Fundamentals of Anaesthesia and Acute Medicine

Preoperative Assessment

FUNDAMENTALS OF ANAESTHESIA AND ACUTE MEDICINE

Series editors

Ronald M Jones, Professor of Anaesthetics, St Mary's Hospital Medical School, London, UK
Alan R Aitkenhead, Professor of Anaesthetics, University of Nottingham, UK
Pierre Foëx, Nuffield Professor of Anaesthetics, University of Oxford, UK

Titles already available:

Anaesthesia for Obstetrics and Gynaecology
Edited by Robin Russell

Cardiovascular Physiology (second edition)
Edited by Hans Joachim Priebe and Karl Skarvan

Clinical Cardiovascular Medicine in Anaesthesia
Edited by Pierre Coriat

Day Care Anaesthesia
Edited by Ian Smith

Intensive Care Medicine
Edited by Julian Bion

Local and Regional Anaesthesia
Edited by Per Rosenberg

Management of Acute and Chronic Pain
Edited by Narinder Rawal

Neuro-Anaesthetic Practice
Edited by H Van Aken

Neuromuscular Transmission
Edited by Leo HDJ Booij

Paediatric Intensive Care
Edited by Alan Duncan

Forthcoming:

Pharmacology of the Critically Ill
Edited by Maire Shelly and Gilbert Park

Fundamentals of Anaesthesia and Acute Medicine

Preoperative Assessment

Edited by

Jeremy N Cashman
Consultant Anaesthetist, St George's Hospital, London, UK

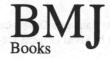

BMJ
Books

© BMJ Books 2001
BMJ Books is an imprint of the BMJ Publishing Group

All rights reserved. No part of this publication may be reproduced,
stored in a retrieval system, or transmitted, in any form or by any
means, electronic, mechanical, photocopying, recording and/or
otherwise, without the prior written permission of the publishers.

First published in 2001
by BMJ Books, BMA House, Tavistock Square,
London WC1H 9JR
www.bmjbooks.com

British Library Cataloguing in Publication Data
A catalogue record for this book is available from the
British Library

ISBN 0-7279-1479-0

Cover design by Landmark Design, Croydon, Surrey
Typeset by Saxon Graphics Ltd, Derby

Contents

Contributors   vi

Foreword to the Fundamentals of Anaesthesia and Acute
Medicine Series   vii
RONALD M JONES, ALAN R AITKENHEAD, PIERRE FOËX

Preface   ix
JEREMY N CASHMAN

Section 1: Preoperative assessment of the patient

1   The preoperative visit   3
    JEREMY N CASHMAN

2   History and examination   21
    RODNEY F ARMSTRONG

3   Preoperative investigations   35
    JOSEPH FOSS

4   Implications of intercurrent disease   58
    LESLEY M BROMLEY

Section 2: Risk assessment

5   Assessing risk   79
    JEAN-PIERRE VAN BESOUW

Section 3: Preoperative preparation of the patient

6   Preoperative optimisation   93
    VERGHESE T CHERIAN, ANDREW A TOMLINSON

7   Patient consent   133
    CHRISTOPHER HENEGHAN

8   Preoperative fasting   149
    SARAH YOUNG, STEPHANIE PHILLIPS

9   Premedication   164
    CARL GWINNUTT, ANTHONY MCCLUSKEY

Epilogue   185
Index   186

Contributors

Rodney F Armstrong
Consultant Anaesthetist, The Middlesex & University College Hospitals, London, England

Lesley M Bromley
Senior Clinical Lecturer, University College London Medical School, London, England

Jeremy N Cashman
Consultant Anaesthetist, St George's Hospital, London, England

Verghese T Cherian
Consultant Anaesthetist, CMC Hospital, Vellore, India

Joseph Foss
Professor of Anesthesiology, University of Chicago, Chicago, USA

Carl Gwinnutt
Consultant Anaesthetist, Hope Hospital, Salford, England

Christopher Heneghan
Consultant Anaesthetist and Barrister at Law, Neville Hall Hospital, Abergavenny, Wales

Anthony McCluskey
Consultant Anaesthetist, Stepping Hill Hospital, Stockport, England

Stephanie Phillips
Consultant Anaesthetist, Sydney Adventist Hospital, Sydney, Australia

Andrew A Tomlinson
Consultant Anaesthetist, North Staffordshire Hospital, Stoke-on-Trent, England

Jean-Pierre van Besouw
Consultant Anaesthetist, St George's Hospital, London, England

Sarah Young
Provisional Fellow, Westmead Hospital, Sydney, Australia

Foreword to the Fundamentals of Anaesthesia and Acute Medicine series

The pace of change within the biological sciences continues to increase and nowhere is this more apparent than in the specialties of anaesthesia, acute medicine, and intensive care. Although many practitioners continue to rely on comprehensive but bulky texts for references, the accelerating rate of biomedical advances makes this source of information increasingly likely to be dated, even if the latest edition is used, The series *Fundamentals of Anaesthesia and Acute Medicine* aims to bring to the reader up-to-date with authoritative reviews of the principal clinical topics which make up the specialties. Each volume will cover the fundamentals of the topic in a comprehensive manner but will also emphasise recent developments or controversial issues.

International differences in the practice of anaesthesia and intensive care are now much less than in the past and the editors of each volume have commissioned chapters from acknowledged authorities throughout the world to assemble contributions of the highest possible calibre. Three volumes will appear annually and, as the pace and extent of clinically significant advances varies among the individual topics, new editions will be commissioned to ensure that practitioners will be in a position to keep abreast of the important developments within the specialties.

Not only does the pace of advance in biomedical science serve to justify the appearance of an international series of this nature but the current awareness of the need for more formal continuing education also underlines the timeliness of its appearance. The editors would welcome feedback from readers about the series, which is aimed at both established practitioners and trainees preparing for degrees and diplomas in anaesthesia and intensive care.

RONALD M JONES
ALAN R AITKENHEAD
PIERRE FOËX

Preface

JEREMY N CASHMAN

The preparation of the patient ... requires no special comment.

Goodman-Levy A. 1922[1]

Introduction

This book is devoted to assessment and preparation of the patient for anaesthesia and surgery. This is a subject which until relatively recently has been somewhat undervalued, with few (mainly observational) studies of the effect of preoperative patient evaluation on patient outcome. Yet the overall safety of modern anaesthesia is a tribute to the efforts of anaesthetists in minimising risks. Fifty years ago the incidence of anaesthesia-related death (death in which anaesthesia played a primary or contributory role) in 10 institutions in the USA was 1:1500.[2] Nearly 40 years later this figure was not changed markedly, at 1:1700.[3] However, at the time (late 1980s) in only 1:10 000 of cases was death totally the result of the anaesthetic.[3] The most recent figures indicate that mortality attributable solely to anaesthesia (anaesthesia-induced death) lies between 1:68 000[4] and 1:185 000[5] for in-hospital patients. Furthermore, occurrence screening has revealed that despite major differences across hospitals with regard to patient casemix, workload, anaesthetic drugs, and monitoring, the rates of major events and deaths were similar.[6]

In the past the question was posed of whether or not a patient in poor physical condition would survive an anaesthetic. Nowadays it is the quality of pre-, peri- and postanaesthetic care that largely determines whether outcome will be satisfactory. Preoperative evaluation should aim to assess the patient's preoperative state, diagnose and then correct, or at least optimise, any diseases or abnormalities relevant to the subsequent anaesthetic. However, preoperative assessment poses challenges for the anaesthetist from a number of perspectives, not the least of these being from clinical and organisational points of view. Thus, as the Audit Commission in the UK has highlighted,[7] one of the challenges facing anaesthetists is that they need to be able to acquire the necessary information about their patients to decide if they are fit for surgery and, if not, what might be done to achieve fitness.

Whilst this book does not set out to provide didactic guidelines for how to deal with every patient, it does aim to provide the reader with a thorough understanding of the issues involved in ensuring that their patient arrives in the operating theatre suite in the best possible physical and mental condition. The book can be read in three discrete sections, although it is inevitable in a book of this type that there will be a degree of overlap between chapters. The first four chapters consider the purposes and the mechanism of the preoperative visit, the approach to obtaining a history from and examination of patients and the adequacy of preoperative testing and how to devise suitably comprehensive test programmes. The difficult topic of the implications of intercurrent disease is also considered. The history obtained, together with physical examination of the patient and the results of subsequent special investigations should alert the anaesthetist to potential problems that may threaten a patient's safety. In addition, an anaesthetic testing programme can be devised that makes suggestions for which tests are required in elective cases as well as those tests indicated by elucidation of symptoms and from examination of the patient. However, whilst there is justifiable concern to avoid the unindicated ordering of invasive investigations or diagnostic procedures, it should be borne in mind that under-ordering of tests is associated with its own dangers.[8] For example, the 12-lead electrocardiogram (ECG) is one test which has become routine but it would seem that due to the occurrence of false positives,[9] age 50+ years is an appropriate cut-off point for ECG screening for patients without known risk factors.[10] The next chapter addresses the important topic of analysis of risk assessment. In particular, the influence of cardiovascular and respiratory disease has been extensively studied. This chapter provides the link between the first four chapters and the last four chapters. The remaining four chapters deal with the overall preparation of patients for anaesthesia and surgery. Preoperative optimising of the patient, obtaining valid consent, ensuring that an adequate duration of fasting and that appropriate premedication has been prescribed are all considered in detail. Preoperative optimisation of the patient is the process of making sure that the patient's medical condition, if any, is adequately controlled. It is important that valid consent has been obtained. How we obtain valid consent, and indeed what we should tell them, is presented in a manner that can be understood by all. Current views on the correct duration of preoperative fasting are coming under increasing scrutiny. The issues involved are addressed and the various different national guidelines are presented. The final chapter addresses the important topic of pharmacological premedication. This subject has seen some of the greatest change in anaesthetists' practice. The chapter provides advice that will ensure that appropriate premedication is prescribed.

1   Goodman-Levy A. *Chloroform anaesthesia*. London: John Bale, Sons and Danielsson, 1922: 136.
2   Beecher HK, Todd DP. A study of the deaths associated with anaesthesia and surgery. Based on a study of 599, 548 anaesthesias in ten institutions 1948–1952, inclusive. *Ann Surg* 1954; 140; 2–35.

3   Lunn JN, Mushin WW. *Mortality associated with anaesthesia.* London: Nuffield Provincial Hospitals Trust, 1982.
4   ANZCA Working Party on Anaesthetic Mortality. *Anaesthesia related mortality in Australia 1991–93.* Melbourne: ANZCA, 1998.
5   Lunn JN, Devlin HB. Lessons from the Confidential Enquiry into Perioperative Deaths in three NHS regions. *Lancet* 1987; **ii**: 1384–6.
6   Cohen MM, Duncan PG, Pope WD *et al.* The Canadian four-centre study of anaesthetic outcomes: can outcomes be used to assess the quality of anaesthetic care? *Can J Anaesth* 1992; **39**: 430–9.
7   Audit Commission. *Anaesthesia under examination.* London: Audit Commission, 1997.
8   Roizen MF, Foss JF, Fischer SP. Preoperative evaluation. In: Miller R, ed. *Anesthesia,* Vol II, 5th edn. New York: Churchill Livingstone, 1999: 824–83.
9   Cashman J, Murdoch L, Kerr L, Haywood G, Shearer R. The value of the preoperative ECG as risk separator before transurethral prostatectomy. *Br J Anaesth* 1997; **78** (suppl 1): A8.
10   Gold BS, Young ML, Kinman JL, Kitz DS, Berlin J, Senford-Schwartz J. The utility of preoperative electrocardiograms in the ambulatory surgical patient. *Arch Intern Med* 1992; **1152**: 301–5.

SECTION 1: Preoperative assessment of the patient

1: The preoperative visit

JEREMY N CASHMAN

"They pour sleep on their head,
And sit down by their bed."

Night, William Blake (1757–1827)

Introduction

The ideal anaesthetic management consists of the preanaesthetic attainment of a state in which a diagnostic procedure, therapeutic procedure or an operation can be performed with as little physiological and psychological trauma to the patient as possible.[1] The preoperative visit is an opportunity for the anaesthetist to meet with his or her patient and discuss with them their anaesthetic. As such, it is an integral part of every anaesthetic. Intuitively, anaesthetists may feel that the preoperative visit, with its one-to-one consultation between anaesthetist and patient, must be of benefit to the patient. Thus it has been proposed that the preoperative visit might have a therapeutic effect and may even be useful in reducing patients' anxiety.[2] However, it is difficult to identify randomised controlled clinical trials that have investigated specifically the beneficial effect on anaesthetic outcome of the preanaesthetic evaluation.

There have been many changes in anaesthetic practice over recent years that have caused us to review our approach to the preoperative visit. This chapter will address preoperative screening as well as preoperative assessment and evaluation.

The preoperative visit: current practice

Every patient scheduled for anaesthesia and surgery should be evaluated by an anaesthetist preoperatively.[3] Such evaluation should occur sufficiently far in advance of any impending surgery to allow for adequate preoperative optimisation. Rarely, in exceptional circumstances (such as acute myocardial ischaemia following failed coronary angioplasty, ruptured aortic aneurysm and so on), it may be acceptable for patients to receive only a cursory evaluation before being assessed on arrival in the anaesthetic room.[1,4] In contrast, increasing workload in the operating theatre[5] cannot be considered an acceptable reason why anaesthetists cannot afford the time to visit patients preoperatively.

There has been a marked change in surgical, and as a result anaesthetic, practice over recent years. More and more operations are being carried out as day case procedures. At the same time there has been a trend for patients undergoing operations performed as inpatient procedures to be admitted to hospital later and later, with the result that there are fewer and fewer (or in extreme cases no) in-hospital presurgery days.[3] As a result, same-day admission even for quite major surgery is common. Currently in the USA approximately 65% of operations are performed as day case procedures and a further 20–30% are performed as morning-of-surgery admission.[3]

These changes have resulted in greater pressure on anaesthetists to perform preoperative evaluation in an ever shorter period of time. In extreme circumstances very rapid preoperative evaluation is necessary as the anaesthetist moves from one case to the next.[3] At least one author has questioned whether or not it is possible to perform an adequate preoperative evaluation in only 5–15 minutes.[3] Indeed, it is salutary to consider that one study has reported that the average time needed by a physician to conduct a comprehensive preoperative assessment (depending on complexity of medical condition) may be of the order of 27 minutes,[6] a figure that is markedly at variance with the time actually spent at the bedside (Box 1.1).[7]

Best practice dictates that, except in emergency situations, the temptation to bring incompletely evaluated and untreated patients to the anaesthetic room should be resisted.[1] Fortunately, published data seem to indicate that this is indeed the case. In The Netherlands, 'most' patients receive a preoperative visit from their anaesthetist.[8] In a survey conducted in Germany, 98.6% of respondent hospitals prepared their patients with a preoperative visit and anxiolytic premedication[9] whilst in the United Kingdom the 1992–93 NCEPOD report stated that 94% of patients were visited by an anaesthetist before their operation[10] and that the visiting anaesthetist was present at the subsequent operation in 96% of cases. In contrast, over 30% of patients were not visited by a surgeon before their operation. The 1992–93 NCEPOD report speculated that a preoperative visitation rate of 100% was not possible because of true emergencies. The NCEPOD observations contrast with the subsequent findings of the Audit

Box 1.1 Amount of time spent by anaesthetist with patient preoperatively[7]

Not visited	18%
1–5 mins	14%
6–10 mins	35%
11–20 mins	26%
21–30 mins	6%
>30 mins	1%

Commission who reported that one-third of patients either do not meet their anaesthetist before arrival in the operating theatre or do so for only a few minutes.[7]

The purpose of the preoperative visit: screening versus assessment

A substantial proportion of patients presenting for surgery, possibly as many as two-fifths, have severe medical disease in addition to their surgical problem. Of these, the medical condition of nearly 8% can be improved before they are anaesthetised.[11] It is therefore critical for patients to be seen and adequate steps taken to optimise such patients preoperatively. Elderly patients in particular require a thorough evaluation of their perioperative risk[12] with particular attention directed towards cardiac and respiratory status.[13]

Screening

Preoperative screening is the process that ensures that patients are *prima facie* fit for anaesthesia and surgery and that all appropriate investigations are available at the time of the preoperative assessment (Box 1.2). Preoperative screening does not decrease the need for an anaesthetist to visit the patient. Preoperative *screening* can be conducted by nursing staff, other medical staff or anaesthetists. In contrast, preoperative *assessment* is the sole responsibility of the anaesthetist, ideally the one who will administer the anaesthetic.

A number of approaches to screening have been employed, ranging from questionnaires which may be completed by the patient, a nurse or medical staff, anaesthetic or otherwise. The use of preoperative screening in the evaluation of patients prior to anaesthesia and operation is the subject of more detailed texts.[6,12,14,15]

Box 1.2 Aims of preoperative screening

- To provide the anaesthetist with basic information on the patient's health status which will enable a meaningful assessment of fitness for anaesthesia to be made
- To identify and instigate relevant investigations according to predetermined protocols
- To increase the patient's understanding of pre-, intra- and postoperative care

And specifically in the case of day stay surgery:

- To assess home situation, social circumstances, and availability of support

---

5

The preanaesthetic assessment clinic

Preoperative anaesthetic screening and assessment clinics were developed as a response to morning-of-operation admission, with the associated reduction in time available for assessment and effecting improvement in the patients prior to surgery. The preadmission assessment of patients 1–2 weeks preoperatively has now become the standard across North America.[16-19] Such clinics are now considered highly effective and most anaesthetic departments issue written guidelines detailing which patients should be referred.[16,17,19]

A variety of structures for preanaesthetic assessment clinics have been developed, ranging from those that employ full-time trained nurses to staffing by as-available anaesthetists. The most common model for preoperative screening clinics is one in which patients are seen and assessed by a nurse who decides on onward referral to an anaesthetist. Refinements to this system include the use of a preoperative questionnaire as a tool to aid screening. Patients are only assessed by an anaesthetist if they have a positive questionnaire or if referred direct by their surgeon.[17-18] In this latter context the preoperative questionnaire is invaluable as an initial screening tool, since surgeons may not always be aware of the full medical history or potential anaesthetic risks.[18] Furthermore, it is uncommon for patients to be preassessed by an anaesthetist on the same day as they are seen by their surgeon,[17] an approach which might have potential advantages.

Another advantage of preanaesthetic assessment clinics is that immediate onward referral for specialist physician opinion may be available. This is especially important with regard to diseases of the cardiovascular and respiratory systems. In one survey, access to a cardiological opinion was available in nearly a third of clinics.[17]

Methods of preanaesthetic assessment
A detailed history and full medical examination are considered to be the most effective way to screen for disease. Specific investigations and tests are used to confirm clinical diagnosis and aid in optimising the patient.

Preanaesthetic assessment questionnaires can be used for patients to indicate details of any relevant medical condition or previous anaesthetic problems.[20] The information obtained can then reviewed by a specially trained nurse who can, in addition, record details of current medication and decide on the advisability of anaesthetic review. Screening questionnaires have been criticised for employing a broad-sweep approach that merely collects patient information and links it to a blanket recommendation for further investigations. However, preoperative anaesthetic assessment questionnaires which focus on those patients at risk have been designed.[18] Thus, in a comparison of "individual" screening versus "routine" preoperative screening programmes, Christian and colleagues found that non-selective

6

routine screening, although having a relatively high pick-up rate, was not sufficiently sensitive to be economically reasonable.[14] (See also Chapter 3.)

The development of computerised automation in preoperative screening has resulted in the design of patient-completed screening questionnaires that can be scanned electronically into a database which is programmed to trigger further assessment according to a preset algorithm.[15] The computer-interpreted screening questionnaire approach compares favourably with nurse screening or indeed nurse interpretation of screening questionnaires.

Complete automation is afforded by programmes such as HealthQuiz[21] (website www.healthquiz.com). In this approach the patient interacts directly with a computer which elicits a history and suggests appropriate laboratory tests. The HealthQuiz approach has been found to be as good as conventional doctor/patient interview[21] but does not necessarily save time or resources.[6]

Who should conduct the preoperative assessment?

Assessment by nurses

Nurses can be employed to document relevant information and check that all appropriate stages in the preoperative pathway have been completed. They can also educate the patient with regard to the procedure and what to expect before, during and after surgery. After all relevant information has been gathered and reviewed, complicated patients are referred on to a clinician. More straightforward patients are not seen by an anaesthetist until the immediate preoperative interview. This approach, whereby a trained assessment nurse performs initial screening, has been most successful in day case surgery screening[22] but is also common for inpatient preanaesthetic screening. The patient's surgeon is the commonest source of referral, with 46% of patients referred on to an anaesthetist for additional review before the day of surgery, the remainder being assessed by the anaesthetist on the day of surgery. Of those patients referred to the assessment clinic, 51% were also seen by a physician at first screening.[16]

It should always be remembered that it is inappropriate for a non-anaesthetist to promise a particular type of premedication, anaesthetic technique or postoperative pain management.

Assessment by doctors

Current practice in most UK centres is for patients to be seen preoperatively by both anaesthetist and surgeon. However, in some hospitals the patient is "cleared" for surgery by a junior member of the surgical team following discussion with an anaesthetist. In his or her assessment of the patient, the junior surgical trainee is primarily concerned with the patient's fitness for the operation as well as the specific condition to be treated whereas the anaesthetist is concerned with whether or not the patient is fit for an anaesthetic. Banerjee and colleagues, in questioning whether or not this duplication in preoperative assessment was necessary, found little overlap.[23] There was a low level of disagreement between anaesthetist and surgeon which was only 9% greater than by chance. This is not surprising since surgeons are not always aware of the full medical history or potential anaesthetic risks.[17]

Cardiology opinions are often requested by surgeons, and by anaesthetists, for patients with cardiovascular disease. However, there is often confusion regarding the exact reason for the referral and its implication for patient management. Furthermore, there is substantial disagreement between all involved (anaesthetist, cardiologist, and surgeon) on the importance and purpose of the referral.[24] Most surgeons felt obliged to follow a cardiologist's recommendations whereas few anaesthetists felt so obliged. The authors of the survey (themselves anaesthetists!) concluded that most cardiology consultations gave little advice that truly affected patient management.[24]

Assessment by an anaesthetist

The American Society of Anesthesiologists has laid out basic standards for preanaesthetic care, including preoperative evaluation.[25] These state that although various non-anaesthetic personnel may gather and correlate information, the final responsibility for determining the medical status of the patient and developing and discussing with the patient a plan of anaesthetic care rests with the anaesthetist. In a detailed review, Klafta and Roizen observe that the preoperative consultation by an anaesthetist has six purposes (Box 1.3).[26]

The preoperative evaluation of the surgical patient enhances the anaesthetist's awareness of the patient's medical condition and facilitates planning of perioperative care. Many studies attest to the importance of a carefully taken history, a meticulous physical examination, and the preoperative performance of specific screening tests.[14]

A thorough preanaesthetic evaluation is important in preventing anaesthetic morbidity and mortality and ensuring a smooth course of anaesthetic

Box 1.3 Purpose of preoperative consultation by an anaesthetist[3]

- To assess and ensure readiness of patients for anaesthesia and surgery
- To choose the anaesthetic and educate the patient regarding the planned technique
- To reassure the patient and decrease anxiety
- To discuss postoperative care
- To decrease costs by improving outcome and reducing length of stay
- To obtain consent for specific aspects of anaesthesia

---

administration.[27] Indeed, the patient's preoperative disease is often predictive of intraoperative events relating to the same organ system.[28] Thus the preoperative medical assessment provides an opportunity for the anaesthetist to gain the patient's confidence and to reduce perioperative morbidity by optimising preoperative status and planning perioperative management. Consultation consists of introduction and interview, with a chance to allay the patient's anxiety, an evaluation of the history, thorough physical examination, and interpretation of data from specific investigations. Finally an explanation of the procedure, its associated risks and the alternative options (for example, general versus regional anaesthetic techniques) may be given.

An anaesthetic-orientated history and examination should focus on those organ systems which are most obviously affected by anaesthetics or which themselves exert an influence on the course of anaesthesia and the postoperative period. Evaluation of acute and/or chronic disease in addition to the surgical lesion is also important. Thus the history should focus on disorders of the cardiovascular, respiratory, central nervous, metabolic, and hepatorenal systems. Previous anaesthetic experience, drug history (current and previous medication as well as allergic disposition), smoking, and drinking habits should be elicited. In the physical examination, attention should be paid to the cardiovascular and respiratory systems, inspection of head and neck, and examination for possible airway problems (Box 1.4).

It has been shown that anaesthetists exhibit a high degree of accuracy in their preoperative diagnosis of co-existing disease which may make anaesthesia and operation excessively risky. Furthermore, in such cases, ignoring the anaesthetists' suggestions for modification of preoperative medical management has been shown to be associated with a significantly higher complication rate (33.2% versus 18.1%) and, indeed, mortality (2.3% versus 5.2%).[11]

In one study information that significantly altered the subsequent anaesthetic management was discovered in 15% of patients. However, in less than 3% of cases would ignorance of the patient's condition have required postponement of surgery.[29] The authors of this study concluded that the major reason for the preoperative visit by an anaesthetist was that patients appreciated it rather than it being medically necessary! Finally, patients may not remember what they have been asked at the preoperative visit.[29]

Psychological preparation

Despite a wide variation in patients' perception of the importance of the preoperative visit, it is apparent that the majority of patients attach great importance to the preoperative consultation with their anaesthetist. Meeting the anaesthetist preoperatively was the highest priority of patients in the study by Lonsdale and colleagues.[30] Patient factors (such as age, gender, etc.), previous anaesthetic experiences and the nature of the

Box 1.4 Preoperative assessment questionnaire

- Name   Age   Weight   Height (body mass index)
- Proposed operation
- Previous anaesthetic history
- Own or family (blood relative) history of anaesthetic complication
- Dentition – own, crowns, loose
- Allergies – drugs, foods, contact, other
- Smoker – cigarette, pipe
- Alcohol intake – units per week
- History of :

Chest pain	Asthma	Diabetes	Seizures	Heartburn
Heart disease	Bronchitis	Hepatitis/jaundice	Blackouts	Hiatus hernia
High blood pressure	TB	Bleeding problems	Stroke/TIA	Peptic ulcer
Palpitations	Dyspnoea		Muscle	
Exertional dyspnoea			weakness	
Orthopnoea			Psychiatric	
Other medical conditions (including cancer)			illness	

- Pregnant?
- Current medication including OCP, aspirin, etc.
- Any relevant beliefs, religious or otherwise

TB, tubercullosis; TIA, transient ischaemic attack; OCP, oral contraceptive pill

impending surgery all have an important bearing on the patient's perception of the preoperative visit. Age is inversely related to degree of concern, whilst female patients express more fears regarding their anaesthetic.[26] However, there are contrasting views regarding the importance of previous anaesthetic experience. Klafta and Roizen noted a lack of correlation between anxiety and prior anaesthetic experience[26] whereas Tolksdorf reported a link between quality of previous anaesthetic experience and anxiety.[31] Furthermore, Tolksdorf noted that surgical factors, in particular a diagnosis of cancer, increased preoperative anxiety.[31]

Patients often express a desire to be given full and comprehensive details of the complications of anaesthesia and surgery but simply providing information to patients does not decrease anxiety unless the information increases the patient's perception of control.[32] Paradoxically patients, although keen to receive preoperative information, seem to be more interested in postoperative landmarks such as resumption of eating and drinking than hearing about dangerous complications of anaesthesia and surgery.[30]

Patients' anxiety and fears

Anxiety can be considered as being of two distinct types. Trait (or dispositional) anxiety is the level of anxiety inherent in the individual while state (or situational) anxiety is the level of anxiety induced by environmental factors. Trait anxiety is unchanged by events such as impending surgery but state anxiety may dramatically increase. Patients with inherently high trait anxiety tend to react with a greater increase in state anxiety in the perioperative period.[33] State and trait anxiety levels can be measured using the Spielberger Stait/Trait Inventory (STAI).[33] As anaesthetists in general are poor judges of anxiety,[34,35] tools such as the STAI, Hospital Anxiety and Depression (HAD) Scale, Multiple Affect Adjective Checklist (MAACL) and even visual analogue scales, all of which are equivalent,[36] should be used routinely for measurement of anxiety.

There are a multitude of factors associated with high preoperative anxiety levels. These include lack of previous anaesthetic/surgical experience and female gender. The position on the operating list (beginning or later) may also affect the level of anxiety.[37] Removal of dentures also contributes to the preoperative distress of patients.[38]

It is a commonly held view that the patient's anxiety peaks in the period immediately prior to surgery. This may not necessarily be the case. In one study only a small percentage of patients reached their peak level of anxiety on the morning of surgery.[39] Indeed, anxiety levels may be highest in the first few days immediately after surgery.[40] It has been suggested that a high level of preoperative anxiety does have implications for patients' subsequent progress and that anxiety on the afternoon before surgery can predict anxiety in the immediate preoperative period.[34,41] Thus assessment at this time may allow prescription of appropriate anxiolytic premedication. In contrast, another study was unable to find any correlation between anxiety scores on the evening before surgery and those on the morning of operation.[37]

Why decrease anxiety?
Anxiety can adversely affect physiological parameters before and during anaesthesia.[42,43] In addition, preoperative anxiety can affect postoperative course, including morbidity and duration of hospitalisation. In particular, increased preoperative anxiety is associated with increased postoperative pain.[44,47]

How to decrease anxiety
Patients have fears about the anaesthetic that are distinct from their fears concerning their surgery.[8,27] More than a third of patients are afraid of the anaesthetic as distinct from the surgery.[9] The preanaesthetic visit has traditionally been considered to have a beneficial effect on anxiety whether this is conducted by an anaesthetist[45] or a member of the theatre nursing team.[46] A frank preoperative discussion may be all that is necessary to allay anxiety in many patients.[45]

Having assessed the patient's level of anxiety, the anaesthetist is then in a position to try to reduce it. There are two types of preparation for surgery: information preparation and coping preparation.[33] The perception of having control over a situation rather than being well informed determines the patient's level of stress. Excessive information may serve to

11

increase anxiety, at least initially. Preoperative information booklets are simple and easy to implement. However, patients' coping behaviour varies considerably and strongly influences the usefulness of providing preoperative information.[27] This may explain the conflicting reports of the effectiveness of such information booklets.[5,47] Although pharmacological anxiolysis has been the mainstay of attempts to decrease anxiety (See Chapter 9), other techniques have been described. At present, psychological methods of preoperative preparation (including counselling and other approaches such as biofeedback and relaxation techniques) are not routinely used.[9]

The preoperative visit can have other important consequences. Thus, the anaesthetist's appearance might be a factor. One study has reported that although patients preferred traditional attire, paradoxically the clothing worn by an anaesthetist seemed irrelevant to the patient's satisfaction.[48] Finally good communication with patients not only results in an improved rapport but is also associated with a lower incidence of malpractice litigation.[26]

Other considerations

In addition to evaluation of the patient's anxiety, it may be necessary to assess a number of other aspects of their condition and history.

Nutrition

Nutritional status is particularly important in patients with diagnoses such as Crohn's disease in which they are likely to be or to become malnourished.[48–50] Obesity also poses substantial risks. Thus both obesity and malnutrition are associated with a higher incidence and greater severity of perioperative adverse effects. There is a U-shaped association between weight and perioperative adverse events. Extreme over- and underweight are associated with a greater incidence of adverse effects (38%) than mild-to-moderate over- and underweight (31% and 36% respectively). The lowest incidence of adverse effects (23%) occurs in patients of normal weight.[51] In addition, obesity and inadequate fasting are associated with greater recovery problems.[28] The topic of preoperative fasting is discussed in Chapter 8.

Drugs in the perioperative period

Many patients admitted to hospital for operation will be taking medication which may affect or be affected by the drugs used during anaesthesia. The most commonly encountered classes of drugs which patients may be taking include α_2-adrenoceptor and β-adrenoceptor antagonists, ACE inhibitors, calcium channel blockers, antiarrhythmics (including digoxin), anti-coagulant and antiplatelet drugs, bronchodilators, antidiabetic therapy, steroid/hormone therapy, antacids, and gastrokinetic agents. To reduce the possibility of drug interactions occurring, a full drug history should be taken during the preoperative screening assessment. Dawson and Karalliedde[52] have produced a comprehensive list of drug interactions of relevance to anaesthetists.

The perioperative drug management of patients with diabetes mellitus or those taking corticosteroids,[53] hormone replacement therapy and oral contraceptives[54] or drugs for cardiovacular disease[55] presenting for surgery poses particular challenges. It may be necessary to decide on discontinuation of preoperative medication (Box 1.5).[56] If necessary drug therapy may need to be stopped or adjusted sufficiently in advance of surgery and restarted after surgery as appropriate. A detailed review of current medication should be made together with an assessment of the necessity for continuation in the perioperative period. It may be possible to substitute alternative short-acting or even reversible drugs that can be withheld on the morning of surgery; the short-acting reversible MAOI moclobemide is an example.[56] (See also Chapter 6.)

Box 1.5 Long-term medication in patients undergoing surgery[52-55]

- *Drugs that should be continued*
  Antacid and gastrokinetic agents
  Antiepileptics
  Antihypertensives, antianginal, and antiarrhythmic drugs
  Antiparkinsonian drugs
  Antipsychotics and anxiolytics
  Corticosteroids
  Drugs for asthma
  Drugs of dependence
  Immmunosuppressants
  Selective serotonin reuptake inhibitors

- *Drugs that should be stopped or substituted by alternative agents**
  Anticoagulant and antiplatelet drugs
  Antidiabetic therapy
  Aspirin and other NSAIDS
  Diuretics
  Lithium
  MAOIs
  Oral contraceptives and hormone replacement therapy

---

* There are very few medicines which should be withheld before surgery in order to decrease the risks that they impose on the procedure.

13

Miscellaneous

Educational
Unfortunately for our specialty there is a lack of awareness, not just amongst the general public but also amongst some of our colleagues, concerning the roles and skills of anaesthetists. A recent letter (early 2000) from an eminent professor of cardiological sciences serves as an illustration.

> *"Many thanks for your note. I am pleased that ECG monitoring is now routine here. However, it would be helpful for me to know if ECG monitoring is routine for all general anaesthetics everywhere. I could then save a sentence or two in all similar letters that I write."*

Perhaps it is not surprising therefore that a substantial proportion of the general public (up to 50% in the USA, Australia, and Great Britain) are under the misconception that anaesthetists are not physicians.[26] In one survey conducted in a British hospital, only 65% of patients thought that the anaesthetist was a doctor.[57] Yet despite this finding, confidence in anaesthetists is high! It can only be hoped that initiatives such as the National Anaesthesia Days in Australia, New Zealand, and the UK will help to raise the public's perception of our specialty.

Risk assessment
The preoperative evaluation allows the anaesthetist to identify likely risks of impending anaesthesia and surgery which in turn allow an estimation of the possibility of complications occurring so that he or she can plan steps to reduce or eliminate such an eventuality. The ASA classification has broad predictive value for morbidity and mortality.[58] Risk assessment is covered in more detail in Chapter 5.

Special circumstances

Elective surgery

Scheduled and elective operations account for one-third of all operations in the UK. Preoperative risk factors can be divided into those arising from the environment; the surgeon and the nature of the operative intervention; the nature of the anaesthetic technique; the disease; and the patient's preoperative (premorbid) medical status regardless of current illness.[59] Based on these factors, a schedule for the preparation of patients that can be developed[60] (see also Chapter 3). High-risk patients offer a particular challenge in the preoperative assessment[61] and this is especially true for cardiac patients undergoing non-cardiac surgery.[62,63]

Preoperative assessment of preexisting and chronic disease requires a careful search for local and systemic manifestations of the disease.[50, 58, 60, 64] In particular, preoperative assessment of patients for cardiac surgery must cover specific aspects of the risk entailed. In the case of orthotopic cardiac and lung transplantation, patients will have already received exhaustive counselling including risks of undergoing surgery versus risk of not undergoing surgery. Specific details of preoperative history, diagnosis and the implications of intercurrent disease are covered in Chapters 2 and 4.

Patients with cardiac disease

A detailed assessment of the patient with cardiovascular disease, including history, physical examination and routine investigations, is essential. Fleischer and Barasch have advocated that adherence to the traditional "safe" interval between recent myocardial infarction and surgery could be abandoned in favour of a risk stratification approach.[65] A more recent study which also advocated risk stratification recommends that, in addition to Fleischer and Barasch's risk factors, a history of cerebrovascular disease and an elevated serum creatinine >177 μmol/l are also important patient factors.[66] A subsequent editorial pointed out that 36% of the population have none of these risk factors 39% have one risk factor, 18% have two risk factors, and only 7% have three or more risk factors.[67]

Hypertension is a condition that complicates anaesthetic and postoperative management but which, with appropriate management, should not compromise the patient.[68] Even a simple manoeuvre such as providing information to patients has been shown to have beneficial effects in decreasing the incidence of postoperative hypertension.[32]

Children

There are specific problems relating to the psychological effects of hospitalisation and surgery in children. Approaches to preoperative evaluation and preparation, including psychological preparation of the normal paediatric patient, have been covered in specialised texts including that by Green and McNiece.[69] Preoperative fasting in children is discussed in Chapter 8. The particular challenge posed by the preoperative assessment and subsequent anaesthetic management of the child with a congenital syndrome is addressed by Bevan.[70] In addition, the reader is directed to the list of syndromes with their anaesthetic implications produced by Jones and Pelton.[71]

Jehovah's Witnesses

There are over 5 million active Jehovah's Witnesses throughout the world with close on another 10 million people who might be expected to share some beliefs.[72] The legal position on the management of Jehovah's Witness patients with respect to anaesthesia and consent has been outlined in a

15

booklet produced by the Association of Anaesthetists of Great Britain and Ireland.[72]

There is an increased risk of morbidity and mortality associated with surgery in Jehovah's Witness patients.[73] Hence detailed preoperative assessment is necessary along with pretreatment reassurance that their religious beliefs will be respected regardless of circumstances.[74,75] Such preoperative agreement should be viewed as binding. The situation with regard to children is more complex (see Chapter 7).

Day stay

The specific demands of day stay surgery were the impetus for the development of preanaesthetic screening clinics so it is not surprising that this is a particularly well-developed area. Selection of patients for admission on the day of surgery should conform to locally agreed guidelines, with patients fully assessed and investigated preoperatively at the outpatient visit.[76] Timing of admission on day of surgery should allow final clinical assessment by both surgeon and anaesthetist.

It has been suggested that day case surgery is particularly amenable to the use of routine screening questionnaires.[77] It has also been noted that preoperative assessment for day case surgery carried out by a trained assessment nurse resulted in fewer cancellations, reduced postoperative problems, and more satisfied patients.[23]

In general, only ASA class I and II patients tend to be considered for day stay surgery although there is a trend for more "at-risk" patients to be operated upon as an outpatient procedure.[78] Day stay surgery on patients with preoperative medical conditions, even when optimally managed, is associated with a higher risk for adverse events in the perioperative period.[28] This contrasts with the observations of Kvalsvik, who suggested that many ASA III and even some ASA IV patients can be suitable candidates for day stay surgery.[79]

Emergency surgery

In the UK the degree of urgency of operations has remained reasonably constant over a number of years. Approximately two-fifths of operations are classified as urgent (operation not on a routine operating list but in a patient fully resuscitated) and a further quarter classified as emergency (resuscitation simultaneous with surgical treatment; operation usually within one hour)[80] (Box 1.6).

Surgery may be necessary in the face of co-existing disease, in particular pulmonary and cardiovascular disease and the presence of other disease states such as diabetes mellitus. Assessment of circulating volume should be considered; intravascular volume depletion may be due to acute haemorrhage, burns, third-space losses or dehydration secondary to vomiting, polyuria or other causes.

Box 1.6 1994–95 NCEPOD classification of operation[80]

Emergency	26%
Urgent	41%
Scheduled	22%
Elective	10%

Strict Advanced Trauma Life Support (ATLS) protocols have been developed to assist in dealing with multiple trauma and these should be followed. Thus, eliciting a verbal response from the victim provides an indication of the adequacy of the airway, ventilation, and cerebral perfusion whilst impaired movement of limbs might indicate limb and/or spinal injury. It is important to assess vital signs (Airway, Breathing, Circulation) and to look for signs of shock (tachycardia, pallor, sweating, etc.). It is also important to identify the likely site(s) of trauma. The reader is directed to the ATLS manual.[81]

Conclusion

The preoperative visit serves a highly important function in the preparation of the patient for anaesthesia and surgery. In addition, the preoperative visit may have a therapeutic effect in its own right. However, changes in the working practices of anaesthetists have resulted in the view that the "night before" bedside visit may no longer be tenable. In its place there has been a move to introduce preanaesthetic assessment clinics. Although various models of preanaesthetic assessment clinics have developed, they all have the same objective: evaluating patients sufficiently in advance of surgery to allow optimisation of the patient. The next three chapters will identify those aspects of the patient's history and examination relevant to anaesthesia, assess the value of preoperative investigations with respect to anaesthesia, and consider the implications of abnormalities revealed on history, examination or further investigation.

1   Ashburn MA, Stanley TH. Anesthesiology update: the preanesthetic evaluation. *Compr Ther* 1988; 14: 27–32.
2   Egbert LD, Batti GE, Turndorf H, Beecher HK. The value of the preoperative visit by an anesthetist. *JAMA* 1963; 185: 553–5.
3   Roizen MF, Foss JF, Fischer SP. Preoperative evaluation. In: Miller R, ed. *Anesthesia Volume II*, 5th edn. New York: Churchill Livingstone, 1999: 824–83.
4   AAGBI. *The anaesthesia team*. London: Association of Anaesthetists of Great Britain and Ireland, 1998.
5   Leigh JM, Walker J, Janaganathan P. Effect of preoperative visit on anxiety. *BMJ* 1977; ii: 987–9.
6   Jackson KI, Gibby GL, van der Aa JJ, Arroyo AA, Gravenstein JS. The efficiency of preoperative evaluation: a comparison of computerized and paper recording systems. *J Clin Monit* 1994; 10: 189–93.

17

7   Audit Commission. *Anaesthesia under examination*. London: Audit Comission, 1997.
8   van Wijk MG, Smalhout B. A postoperative analysis of the patient's view of anaesthesia in a Netherlands' teaching hospital. *Anaesthesia* 1990; **45**: 679–82.
9   Roth-Isigkeit A, Schwarzenberger J, Brechmann J, Gehring H, Klotz KF, Schmucker P. Vorbereitung auf elektive eingriffe – Spectrum und verbreitung somatischer und psychologischer massnahmen in Deutschland [The preparation for elective interventions – the spectrum and dissemination of somatic and psychological measures in Germany]. *Anasthesiol Intensivmed Notfallmed* Schmerzther 1997; **32**: 654–8.
10   *The NCEPOD report 1992–93*. London: NCEPOD, 1995.
11   Prause G, Ratzenhofer-Komenda B, Smolle-Juettner F *et al*. Operations on patients deemed "unfit for operation and anaesthesia": what are the consequences? *Acta Anaesthesiol Scand* 1998; **42**: 316–22.
12   van Aken H, Rolf N. Die praoperative evaluierung und vorbereitung. Die sicht des anasthesisten [Preoperative evaluation and preparation. The view of the anaesthetist]. *Anaesthesist* 1997; **46** (suppl. 2): S80–4.
13   Daly MP. The medical evaluation of the elderly preoperative patient. *Prim Care* 1989; **16**: 361–76.
14   Christian KW, Gervais H, Dick W. Aussagewert von praoperativen screeninguntersuchungen [Value of preoperative screening studies]. *Anaesthesist* 1988; **37**: 694–703.
15   Gibby GL, Gravenstein N. Pre-anesthetic evaluation. In: List WF, Metzler H, eds. *Preanaesthetic care*. London: Baillière Tindall, 1998: 503–21.
16   Fischer SP. Development and effectiveness of an anaesthesia preoperative evaluation clinic in a teaching hospital. *Anesthesiology* 1996; **85**: 196–206.
17   Bond DM. Pre-anesthetic assessment clinics in Ontario. *Can J Anaesth* 1999; **46**: 382–7.
18   Badner NH, Craen RA, Paul TL, Doyle JA. Anaesthesia preadmission assessment: a new approach through use of a screening questionnaire. *Can J Anaesth* 1998; **45**: 87–92.
19   Conway JB, Goldberg J, Chung F. Preadmission anaesthesia consultation clinics. *Can J Anaesth* 1992; **39**: 1051–7.
20   Pearson RM, Jago RH. An evaluation of a pre-operative anaesthetic assessment questionnaire. *Anaesthesia* 1981; **36**: 1132–6.
21   Lutner RE, Roizen M, Stocking CB *et al*. The automated interview versus the personal interview. Do patient responses to preoperative health questionnaires differ? *Anesthesiology* 1991; **75**; 394–400.
22   Rudkin GE, Osborne GA, Doyle CE. Assessment and selection of patients for day surgery in a public hospital. *Med J Aust* 1993; **158**: 308–12.
23   Banerjee AR, Reilly PG, Marshall JN, Nunez D. Is pre-operative patient assessment effective? A prospective trial of 100 patients. *Ann R Coll Surg Engl* 1996; **78** (3 suppl.): 119–21.
24   Katz RI, Barnhart JM, Ho G, Hersch D, Dayan SS, Keehn L. A survey on the intended purposes and perceived utility of preoperative cardiology consultations. *Anesth Analg* 1998; **87**: 830–6.
25   American Society of Anesthesiologists. *Basic standards for preanesthetic care*. Park Ridge, Ill: American Society of Anesthesiologists, 1987.
26   Klafta JM, Roizen MF. Current understanding of patients' attitudes toward and preparation for anesthesia: a review. *Anesth Analg* 1996; **83**: 1314–21.
27   Latham LB. Preanesthetic evaluation. *Dent Clin North Am* 1999; **43**: 217–29.
28   Duncan PG, Cohen MM, Tweed WA *et al*. The Canadian four-centre study of anaesthetic outcomes: III. Are anaesthetic complications predictable in day surgical practice? *Can J Anaesth* 1992; **39**: 440–8.
29   Nightingale JJ, Lack JA, Stubbing JF, Reed J. The pre-operative anaesthetic visit. Its value to the patient and the anaesthetist. *Anaesthesia* 1992; **47**: 801–3.
30   Lonsdale M, Hutchison GL. Patients' desire for information about anaesthesia. Scottish and Canadian attitudes. *Anaesthesia* 1991; **46**: 410–12.
31   Tolksdorf W. Das praoperative psychische befinden [The preoperative mental state]. *Fortschr Med* 1984; **102**: 342–5.
32   Anderson EA. Preoperative preparation for cardiac surgery facilitates recovery, reduces psychological distress, and reduces the incidence of acute postoperative hypertension. *J Consult Clin Psychol* 1987; **55**: 513–20.

33 Spielberger CD, Auerbach SM, Wadsworth AP, Dunn TM, Taulbee ES. Emotional reactions to surgery. *J Consult Clin Psychol* 1973; **40**: 33–8.
34 Badner NH, Nielson WR, Munk S, Kwiatkowska C, Gelb AW. Preoperative anxiety: detection and contributing factors. *Can J Anaesth* 1990; **37**: 444–7.
35 Hicks JA, Jenkins JG. The measurement of preoperative anxiety. *J R Soc Med* 1988; **81**: 517–19.
36 Millar K, Jelicic M, Bonke B, Asbury AJ. Assessment of preoperative anxiety: comparison of measures in patients awaiting surgery for breast cancer. *Br J Anaesth* 1995; **74**: 180–3.
37 Panda N, Bajaj A, Pershaud D, Yaddanapud ILN, Chari P. Pre-operative anxiety. Effect of early or late position on the operating list. *Anaesthesia* 1996; **51**: 344–6.
38 Cobley M, Dunne JA, Sanders LD. Stressful pre-operative preparation procedures. The routine removal of dentures during pre-operative preparation contributes to pre-operative distress. *Anaesthesia* 1991; **46**: 1019–22.
39 Johnston M. Anxiety in surgical patients. *Psychol Med* 1980; **10**: 145–52.
40 Vogele C, Steptoe A. Physiological and subjective stress responses in surgical patients. *J Psychosom Res* 1986; **30**: 205–15.
41 Lichtor JL, Johanson CE, Mhoon D, Faure EA, Hassan SZ, Roizen MF. Preoperative anxiety: does anxiety level the afternoon before surgery predict anxiety levels just before surgery? *Anesthesiology* 1987; **67**: 595–9.
42 Tolksdorf W, Schmollinger U, Berlin J, Rey ER. Das praoperative psychische befinden – zusammenhange mit anasthesie – relevanten psychophysiologischen parametern [Preoperative psychological state–correlations with anaesthesia–relevant psychophysiologic parameters]. *Anaesthesiol Intensivther Notfallmed* 1983; **18**: 81–7.
43 Tolksdorf W, Berlin J, Rey ER *et al.* Das praoperative stress. Untersuchung zum verhalten psychischer und physiologischer stressparameter nichtpramedezierter patienten in der praoperativen phase [Preoperative stress. Study of the mental behaviour and parameters of physiological stress in non-premedicated patients during the preoperative period]. *Anaesthesist* 1984; **33**: 212–17.
44 Scott LE, Clum GA, Peoples JB. Preoperative predictors of postoperative pain. *Pain* 1983; **15**: 283–93.
45 Alpert CC, Baker JD, Cooke JE. A rational approach to anaesthetic premedication. *Drugs* 1989; **37**: 219–28.
46 Martin D. Pre-operative visits to reduce patient anxiety: a study. *Nurs Stand* 1996; **10**: 33–8.
47 Wallace LM. Psychological preparation as a method of reducing the stress of surgery. *J Human Stress* 1984; **10**: 62–77.
48 Sanders LD, Gildersleve CD, Rees LT, White M. The impact of the appearance of the anaesthetist on the patient's perception of the pre-operative visit. *Anaesthesia* 1991; **46**: 1056–8.
49 Weiss SM. Nutritional aspects of preoperative management. *Med Clin North Am* 1987; **71**: 369–75.
50 Elliot DL, Tolle SW, Linz DH. Preparing the medically compromised patient for surgery. *Postgrad Med* 1985; **77**: 269–71, 274–5, 278 passim.
51 Schwilk B, Muche R, Bothner U, Brinkmann A, Bartels F, Georgieff M. Zwischenfalle, ereignisse und komplikationen in der perioperativen phase bei normal und fehlernahrten patienten – ergebnisse von 23,056 anasthesien [Incidents, events and complications in the perioperative period in normal and malnourished patients – results of 23,056 patients]. *Anasthesiol Intensivmed Notfallmed Schmerzther* 1995; **30**: 99–107.
52 Dawson J, Karalliedde L. Drug interactions and the clinical anaesthetist. *Eur J Anaesthesiol* 1998; **15**: 172–89.
53 Anon. Drugs in the peri-operative period: 2 – Corticosteroids and therapy for diabetes mellitus. *Drug Ther Bull* 1999; **37**: 68–70.
54 Anon. Drugs in the peri-operative period: 3 – Hormonal contraceptives and hormone replacement therapy. *Drug Ther Bull* 1999; **37**: 78–80.
55 Anon. Drugs in the peri-operative period: 4 – Cardiovascular drugs. *Drug Ther Bull* 1999; **37**: 89–91.
56 Anon. Drugs in the peri-operative period: 1 – Stopping or continuing drugs around surgery. *Drug Ther Bull* 1999; **37**: 62–4.

57 Swinhoe CF, Groves ER. Patients' knowledge of anaesthetic practice and the rôle of anaesthetists. *Anaesthesia* 1994; **49**: 165–6.
58 Menke H, Klein A, John KD, Junginger T. Predictive value of ASA classification for the assessment of the perioperative risk. *Int Surg* 1993; **78**: 266–70.
59 Klotz HP, Candinas D, Largiader F. Praoperative risikoeinschatzung in der elektiven viszeralchirurgie. Studienkonzept-resultate-perspektiven [Preoperative risk assessment in elective visceral surgery. Study design, results, perspectives]. *Langenbecks Arch Chir* 1994; **379**: 341–6.
60 Pasternak LR. Preoperative assessment: guidelines and challenges. *Acta Anaesthesiol Scand* 1997; **111** (suppl): 318–20.
61 Prause G, List WF. Der anaesthesiologische risikopatient. Praoperativen evaluierung, intraoperatives management und postoperative uberwachung [The anesthesiologic risk patient. Preoperative evaluation, intraoperative management and postoperative monitoring]. *Chirurg* 1997; **68**: 775–9.
62 Ford BM, Weich HF, Coetzee AR. Pre-operative assessment of cardiac patients for non-cardiac surgery. *S Afr Med J* 1984; **65**: 235–9.
63 Foex P. Preoperative assessment of patients with cardiac disease. *Br J Anaesth* 1978; **50**; 15–23.
64 Skues MA, Welchew EA. Anaesthesia and rheumatoid arthritis. *Anaesthesia* 1993; **48**: 989–97.
65 Fleisher LA, Barash PG. Preoperative cardiac evaluation for non cardiac surgery: a functional approach. *Anesth Analg* 1992; **74**; 586–98.
66 Lee TH, Marcantonio ER, Mangione CM *et al*. Derivation and prospective validation of a simple index for prediction of cardiac risk of major noncardiac surgery. *Circulation* 1999; **100**: 1043–9.
67 Kellon AD, Banning AP. Is simple clinical assessment adequate for cardiac risk stratification before elective non-cardiac surgery? (commentary) *Lancet* 1999; **354**: 1837–8.
68 Laslett L. Hypertension. Preoperative assessment and perioperative management. *West J Med* 1995; **162**: 215–19.
69 Green MC, McNiece WL. Preoperative evaluation and preparation of the pediatric patient. *Semin Pediatr Surg* 1992; **1**: 4–10.
70 Bevan JC. Congenital syndromes in paediatric anaesthesia: what is important to know. *Can J Anaesth* 1998; **45**: R3–16.
71 Jones AEP, Pelton DA. An index of syndromes and their anaesthetic implications. *Can Anaesth Soc J* 1976; **23**: 207–26.
72 AAGBI. *Management of Anaesthesia for Jehovah's Witnesses*. London: Association of Anaesthetists of Great Britain and Ireland, 1999.
73 Wong DH, Jenkins LC. Surgery in Jehovah's Witnesses. *Can J Anaesth* 1989; **36**: 578–85.
74 Kambouris AA. Major abdominal operations on Jehovah's Witnesses. *Am Surg* 1987; **53**: 350–6.
75 Ashley E. Anaesthesia for Jehovah's Witnesses. *Br J Hosp Med* 1997; **58**: 375–80.
76 *The NCEPOD report 1996–97*. London: NCEPOD, 1998.
77 Rollason WN, Hems G. Preoperative assessment for outpatient anaesthesia. *Ann R Coll Surg* 1981; **63**: 45–9.
78 Griffith KE. Preoperative assessment and preparation. *Int Anesthesiol Clin* 1994; **32**: 17–36.
79 Kvalsvik O, Fourtanier G, Fingerhout A *et al*. Selection of patients for ambulatory surgery. *Tidsskrift for den Norske Laegeforening* 1996; **116**: 500–3.
80 *The NCEPOD report 1994–95*. London: NCEPOD, 1997.
81 American College of Surgeons. *Advanced trauma life support course for physicians*, 5th edn. Chicago: American College of Surgeons, 1993.

2: History and examination

RODNEY F ARMSTRONG

Introduction

During the clinical examination of the surgical patient, the anaesthetist is acting in his or her primary role as a doctor. At the preoperative visit a history and examination should identify any factors that may subsequently threaten the patient's safety. This process requires a review of the notes followed by an uninterrupted examination of the patient at the bedside. The anaesthetist should then be able to focus on, document, and modify those factors that may expose that patient to risk when combined with anaesthesia, surgery, and recovery.

Social, family, and drug history

An awareness of negative social practices such as heavy smoking, alcohol excess or drug dependence is clearly of importance. Smoking has been identified as a cause of increased postoperative morbidity.[1] Its effects include hyperreactivity of the bronchial tree with excessive production of mucus as well as small airway damage. Carbon monoxide levels are elevated and there are deleterious long-term effects on the immune and vascular systems. Stopping smoking preoperatively will result in a fall of carbon monoxide levels after approximately 12 hours, a reduction in sputum volume after several days and a return towards normal ciliary and small airway function after some weeks. Occupational disorders, for example those causing respiratory disease, should also be identified and assessed as part of the system they affect. Family illnesses such as familial hyperlipidaemia and diabetes mellitus (see below) may alert the anaesthetist to unexpected medical conditions. Diabetic patients pose special problems;[2] some experts suggest a fivefold increase in perioperative mortality rate as compared to the non-diabetic patient.

A family history or personal experience of complications from previous anaesthetics should be elicited. Malignant hyperpyrexia is inherited as an autosomal dominant gene.[3] It is a rare disorder of skeletal muscle (1:50 000 to 1:100 000 adult anaesthetics) in which commonly used anaesthetic agents trigger sustained skeletal muscle hypermetabolism. Typically the patient develops tachycardia, tachypnoea, hypercarbia, and acidosis with masseter

21

spasm and generalised muscle rigidity. Rhabdomyolysis, elevated potassium, coagulopathy, and death may result. Treatment with dantrolene and general management of the associated physiological disturbance has been shown to be effective in reducing the mortality rate of this lethal condition.

Plasma cholinesterase (Pche) deficiency is another genetically determined disorder causing anaesthetic problems. Patients who are homozygous for this genetic variant synthesise an abnormal form of cholinesterase incapable of hydrolysing certain muscle relaxants, notably suxamethonium and mivacurium. As a result, a dangerous prolongation of neuromuscular blockade occurs leading to respiratory inadequacy in the immediate postoperative period. Several phenotypes occur in the population so that there may be wide differences in Pche activity and therefore in the duration of extended neuromuscular block. Low Pche activity may also occur in liver and renal failure as well as in the burned patient.

Postoperative nausea and vomiting may be a recurrent problem that can be overcome by preoperative antiemetics, avoidance of opiates and even omission of nitrous oxide in the inspired mixture. Bleeding disorders and tendencies should be considered before epidural or spinal anaesthesia is performed, otherwise postoperative bleeding into the epidural space may cause spinal compression and paraplegia.

Finally a drug history should be taken. Many drugs interact with the anaesthetic process and some, such as anticoagulant therapy, insulin, and some drugs used in psychiatry, can cause significant problems (Table 2.1).

Table 2.1 Drug interactions of relevance to anaesthesia

Drug	Effect
Anticoagulants	Increase bleeding during surgery
	May cause spinal or extradural haematoma
Insulin	Hypoglycaemia during anaesthesia
β-blockers	Bradycardia
MAOIs	Hypertensive response to pressor agents
	React with some opioids
Diuretics	Unrecognised hypokalaemia and arrhythmias
Steroids	Adrenal suppression
Digoxin	Arrhythmias
Calcium channel antagonists	Bradyarrhythmias and decreases in cardiac output
Contraceptive pill	Thromboembolism

MAOI, Monoamine oxidase inhibitor

Cardiovascular system

History

The objective of the cardiovascular assessment is to discover whether the patient has cardiac failure, ischaemia, an arrhythmia, heart murmurs or evidence of poor circulatory function. Key symptoms of cardiac malfunction are:

- breathlessness
- chest pain
- palpitations
- fatigue
- claudication.

Breathlessness on exertion or on lying flat (orthopnoea) is an important indicator of heart failure. Symptoms are produced by a rise in left atrial pressure with pulmonary congestion. Paroxysmal nocturnal dyspnoea suggests pulmonary oedema. When cardiac output fails to provide adequate tissue oxygen delivery, the patient experiences fatigue. The New York Heart Association classification of heart failure provides a more objective description of heart failure (Box 2.1).

Risk factors such as a positive family history of heart disease, diabetes mellitus, smoking, high blood pressure, and hyperlipidaemia should alert the anaesthetist to the possibility of ischaemic heart disease (IHD). Chest pain due to heart disease is typically brought on by exertion, cold weather or anxiety and relieved by rest or nitrates. It is usually constricting in nature and sensed retrosternally with occasional radiation to the arms. Patients will generally know whether or not they have had a previous myocardial infarction. If so, an indication of its severity can be obtained by ascertaining the details of treatment as well as the duration of hospital stay. Non-urgent surgery performed soon after a myocardial infarction is associated with an increased reinfarction rate. For patients who undergo surgery within three

Box 2.1 New York Heart Association (NYHA) classification of heart failure

---

Class
I   Cardiac disease but without resulting limitation of physical activity
  – Ordinary physical activity does not cause undue fatigue, palpitation, dyspnoea or anginal pain
II Cardiac disease resulting in slight limitation of physical activity
  – Comfortable at rest
  – Ordinary physical activity results in fatigue, palpitation, dyspnoea or anginal pain
III Cardiac disease resulting in marked limitation of physical activity
  – Comfortable at rest
  – Less than ordinary physical activity causes fatigue, palpitation, dyspnoea or anginal pain
IV Cardiac disease resulting in inability to carry on any physical activity without discomfort
  – Symptoms of cardiac insufficiency or of anginal syndrome may be present even at rest
  – If any physical activity is undertaken discomfort is increased

---

months of a myocardial infarction, reinfarction rates of 30%, with 50% mortality, have been described. Temporary postponement of surgery in such cases is currently recommended (but see Chapter 6).

Awareness of palpitations or a rapidly beating heart is a useful clue to the presence of arrhythmias and a reminder to review the ECG. This is a good point in the history to check for episodes of syncope due to heart block and to identify pacemaker placement. Apart from the importance of checking the pacemaker position, age and function, it is important to be aware that intraoperative diathermy may affect pacemaker function, leading to arrhythmias. Pacemakers are above all an indication of underlying pathology, usually IHD. For those patients who are pacemaker dependent, the anaesthetist will want to prepare alternatives such as an isoprenaline (isoproterenol) infusion or arrange for an external transcutaneous pacemaker to be present in the operating theatre.

The final part of the cardiovascular history should be directed at the peripheral vascular system. Claudication is the key symptom of peripheral arterial disease and details of distance limitation are helpful in assessing severity. Any increased likelihood of thromboembolism should be noted and questions posed to guide perioperative prophylaxis.[4] Protocols for thromboembolic risk assessment and prophylaxis can be useful as practical guides to management; one such protocol is outlined in Box 2.2. According to this protocol, low-risk patients (total score 0–1) should be treated with antiembolic stockings and early mobilisation. Moderate-risk patients (score 2–3) should receive in addition subcutaneous dalteparin (Fragmin) 2500 units once a day, whilst high-risk patients (score 4+) should receive a higher dose of subcutaneous dalteparin (5000 units od).

Examination

Five important questions need to be answered.

1. Is there any evidence of a low cardiac output or cardiac failure?
2. Is there an arrhythmia?
3. Are there any valvular abnormalities?
4. What is the state of the peripheral blood vessels?
5. Is the blood pressure outside the normal range?

In the presence of left ventricular failure, high pulmonary venous pressure leads to fluid leaking into the alveoli. This causes crackles on examining the bases of the lungs. A third heart sound, gallop rhythm or a tachycardia may be present on auscultation. Tachycardia should not be simply attributed to anxiety. Fever, hypovolaemia, heart failure, and thyroid overactivity may be the cause and if so, need correcting before surgery. Rapid atrial fibrillation, multiple extrasystoles, and tachyarrhythmias also need preoperative treatment, as does heart block.

Box 2.2 Thromboembolic risk assessment and prophylaxis protocol (derived from St George's Hospital Department of Surgery Thromboembolic Prophylaxis Protocol 1999 and reproduced with permission from Harinath G, St John PHM. Use of a thromboembolic risk score to improve thromboprophylaxis in surgical patients. In: *Ann. Roy. Coll. Surg. Engl.*, 1998; **80**: 347–9).

Score 1 for each of:	*Score 2 for each of:*	*Score 3 for each of:*
Age > 40 years	Multiple sclerosis/	Malignant melanoma
Surgery expected to last >30 min	paraplegia	Previous DVT
Expected bedrest > 3 days	Burn >15% total BSA	Planned surgery of
Heart failure		lower limb/pelvis
MI within last 3 months		Trauma
Varicose veins		Known thrombophilic
Use of oral contraceptive pill		state
Pregnancy		
Overweight (BMI >30)		
Previous pelvic or long bone fracture.		

Low risk, total score = 0–1; *Moderate risk*, total score = 2–3; *High risk* total score = 4+.

BSA, body surface area; MI, myocardial infarction; BMI, body mass index; DVT, deep vein thrombosis

Patients with severe heart failure may have cold sweaty hands and peripheral vasoconstriction due to catecholamine secretion. If heart failure has become chronic with right-sided ventricular impairment, there may be evidence of a raised jugular venous pressure and dependent oedema. Examination of the jugular venous pulse may reveal giant *a* waves typical of a stenosed tricuspid valve or hypertrophied right ventricle. Large *v* waves suggest tricuspid regurgitation and cannon waves are a sign of complete heart block.

The presence of a cardiac murmur necessitates further investigations, a cardiological opinion and possibly echocardiography. The vasodilatation and reduction in venous return which is the inevitable consequence of anaesthesia is dangerous in the presence of aortic stenosis or a pericardial effusion as it precipitates acute reductions in venous return and cardiac output. A damaged or abnormal valve may become the site of endocarditis if perioperative antibiotics are omitted.

Hypertension is defined by the World Health Organisation as a blood pressure in excess of 160/90 mmHg. Under anaesthesia the untreated hypertensive patient suffers marked swings in blood pressure which, if severe, may threaten cerebral as well as coronary blood flow. Following anaesthesia the incidence of postoperative infarction or reinfarction is approximately double that of normotensives.[5] Furthermore, retrospective studies of (infrequent) postoperative cardiovascular deaths have demonstrated a strong association with a preoperative history of hypertension.[6] Sustained hypertension and in particular a diastolic pressure in excess of 110 mmHg means that non-urgent surgery may have to be postponed until treatment has started and complications of the disease such as left ventricular failure or renal impairment excluded.

A systolic pressure of less than 100 mmHg or a mean arterial pressure of less than 60 mmHg needs an explanation. Hypovolaemia is not an unusual finding in the average hospital ward and, if unrecognised, will lead to acute and severe hypotension under anaesthesia. Clinical signs and symptoms of hypovolaemia include dry mucous membranes, thirst and dry mouth, cold hands with poorly filled or invisible veins, and low jugular venous pressure. Further clues are provided by evidence of oliguria (<400 ml urine/24 h) and a negative fluid balance on an "intake/output" chart. High plasma and low urinary sodium may reinforce suspicions of a low circulating blood volume and indicate judicious administration of intravenous fluids before surgery is undertaken.

Examination of the radial arteries is a worthwhile step, particularly if intraoperative arterial monitoring is planned. Are they in their correct anatomical position? Is there an alternative blood supply to the hand in the shape of patent ulnar vessels? Chronic arterial insufficiency may be revealed by discoloured or hairless shiny skin or by gangrene of the toes. Signs of hyperlipidaemia such as xanthelasma or a corneal arcus senilus in the younger patient are a warning of coronary artery disease.

Once the history and examination are completed an estimate of cardiac risk can be considered in the light of Goldman's analysis of preoperative risk factors.[7,8] See also Chapter 5.

- Evidence of heart failure
- Recent myocardial infarction
- Arrhythmia
- Premature ventricular contractions
- Major surgery
- Age over 70 years
- Aortic stenosis
- Emergency
- Poor general condition

Although risk estimation is an inexact science it is clear that evidence of increased risk is useful knowledge. For a start, both patient and surgeon can be better informed about likely outcomes. Furthermore, perioperative arrangements such as admitting the patient to a high-dependency bed for preoperative monitoring and/or optimisation[9] are facilitated by recognition that the patient is in a high-risk category.

Respiratory system

History

Given the frequency of postoperative respiratory problems encountered after surgery, it is important to identify those patients particularly at risk.

Key symptoms are:

- dyspnoea
- cough
- sputum
- wheeze.

Dyspnoea or difficulty in breathing is so subjective that further questions are needed to clarify the cause. Exercise tolerance will give an idea of its severity and duration its chronicity. Dyspnoea that changes in intensity from day to day strongly suggests asthma and will indicate specific questions to elucidate trigger factors. Dyspnoea at rest represents a serious anaesthetic challenge and is predictive of a poor respiratory outcome after surgery.[10]

Coughs are a cause for concern. In the young patient they may indicate a hyperresponsive respiratory tract which increases any susceptibility to laryngeal spasm and coughing during induction of anaesthesia.[11] Coughs accompanied by sputum production suggest infection or inflammation further down the airway. Sputum colour is a good guide to the presence of infection which, if present, may be a contraindication to elective surgery. The amount of sputum produced daily is important. If very large, the anaesthetist may prefer to use a regional technique and have an awake patient in order to preserve the cough reflex and allow sputum production throughout the operation.

Some types of cough may point to a specific problem. Coughing after exercise or at night is typical of asthma whilst coughing following meals may indicate aspiration of gastric contents due to oesophageal abnormalities. A barking cough suggests recurrent laryngeal nerve injury.

Wheezing is generally caused by partial bronchial obstruction or by bronchospasm. It may be intermittent, as in asthma, or continuous in the presence of bronchial narrowing. Nocturnal snoring, as in obstructive sleep apnoea, may be a pointer to a difficult airway and is a cause of pulmonary hypertension. As well as a warning to the anaesthetist to prepare for a difficult intubation, it is a reminder to check for signs of impaired right ventricular function, i.e. elevated jugular venous pressure, enlarged liver or oedema of the ankles.

Examination

Examination of the chest follows the usual sequence of inspection, palpation, percussion, and auscultation. Tracheal deviation should be noted and evidence of dullness or hyperresonance to percussion, absence of or added breath sounds should be searched for. In this way bronchospasm, areas of consolidation, collapse, pleural effusions or pneumothorax can be identified. Examination of the hands may reveal clubbing or the tremor and vasodilatation typical of carbon dioxide retention. Cyanosis, dyspnoea at rest, tachypnoea or the use of the accessory muscles of respiration are serious signs of respiratory impairment and contraindicate anaesthesia except in an emergency. Any positive findings are an indication for chest X-ray and arterial blood gas analysis.

Useful bedside measurements suggesting serious impairment of respiratory function are:

- respiratory rate above 30/min
- oxygen saturation <90% on air
- arterial $PaO_2 < 11$ kPa on 40% oxygen
- arterial $PaCO_2$ high enough to reduce the pH below 7.2.

Airway assessment
Fundamental to the process of anaesthesia is control of the airway. During mask anaesthesia a difficult airway can not only result in obstructed breathing and hypoxia but may make intubation difficult or impossible.

Patients with large tongues, bull neck, no teeth, beards, and limited extension of the neck are likely to be difficult to manage with an anaesthetic mask. Intubation difficulties can be predicted to some degree by Mallampati's technique in which the patient is asked to open the mouth and extend the tongue. The visibility of the pillars of the fauces, soft palate, and base of the uvula can then be assessed. Failure to visualise the soft palate suggests a difficult intubation. Other clinical signs associated with potential airway problems are a short thyromental distance (from thyroid notch to mental prominence) of less than 6.5 cm, a receding chin, impaired mandibular protrusion, loss of movement at the atlantooccipital joint, poor mouth opening and prominent incisor teeth. An examination routine is shown in Figure 2.1.

```
              /  Extends?
   Neck    — Bull?
              \  Thyromental distance?


              /  Recedes?
   Chin    — Beard?
              \  Protrudes?


              /  Opens?
   Mouth   — Uvula visible?
              \  Teeth?
```

Figure 2.1 A clinical pathway for assessment of the airway.

Central nervous system

A history of transient ischaemic attacks or cerebrovascular accidents is a predictor of a perioperative stroke. It suggests that cerebral perfusion may be at risk and acts as a reminder to the anaesthetist to maintain a satisfactory mean arterial pressure during anaesthesia. Patients with epilepsy should have a review of their anticonvulsant therapy and an assessment of their seizure frequency and pattern. For elderly patients having day case surgery, it is important to detect dementia or disorientation which may render their return home unsafe.

In the emergency situation and particularly in the hurly burly of the accident and emergency department, careful attention to altered levels of consciousness is necessary in order to avoid anaesthetising injured or drugged patients with unnoticed and deteriorating cerebral function. Unconscious patients should be objectively assessed using the Glasgow Coma Scale (Box 2.3). A score of 15 represents normal brain function. A score of 3 equates with deep coma. Patients scoring less than 8 should usually be intubated for the sake of airway protection and consideration given to possible causes of coma. An early CT scan is usually merited.

Patients with progressive neurological diseases such as multiple sclerosis or motor neurone disease may have muscle wasting. In such cases the administration of depolarising muscle relaxants, for example suxamethonium, can result in dangerous rises in serum potassium levels. Should neurological disease produce a progressive bulbar palsy then protective reflexes may be weakened. Dysarthria and/or dysphagia in these patients should alert the anaesthetist to the possibility of postoperative aspiration of stomach contents when altered laryngeal defence mechanisms are furthur impaired by anaesthetic agents.

Patients suffering from myopathies and dystrophies need careful assessment. These conditions are sometimes associated with cardiomyopathies. When neuromuscular diseases, for example myasthenia gravis, are present there may be an abnormal response to muscle relaxants.

If the respiratory muscles are in any way weakened by neurological disease then it is likely that anaesthesia will produce a temporary worsening of the condition and may precipitate postoperative respiratory failure. Clinical evaluation of respiratory muscle weakness is difficult and objective bedside tests are useful. For example, a vital capacity measurement of less than 1L in a 70 kg male adult is indicative of severe weakness probably necessitating respiratory support.

Abdominal system

A history of heartburn, particularly if associated with bending or lying down, may be suggestive of a hiatus hernia. Aspiration of gastric contents is

29

Box 2.3 The Glasgow Coma Scale

Eyes	Open	Spontaneously	4
		To command	3
		To pain	2
		No response	1
Best motor response	To command	Obeys	6
	To pain	Localises	5
		Flexion withdrawal	4
		Decorticate rigidity	3
		Decerebrate rigidity	2
		No response	1
Best verbal response		Orientated	5
		Disorientated	4
		Inappropriate words	3
		Incomprehensible sounds	2
		No response	1

more common in these patients and should therefore be guarded against by the use of preoperative histamine H_2 blockers (for example, ranitidine), oral sodium citrate, and cricoid pressure at induction. Similar concerns are present in any patient with raised intraabdominal pressure such as the acutely distended abdomen, intestinal obstruction or pregnancy.

The body mass index or Quetelet's index is a useful measurement to make in the larger patient. It is calculated by dividing the patient's weight in kilograms by the square of the height in metres. A patient whose body mass index is greater than 35 is considered to be morbidly obese, a condition associated with serious anaesthetic problems. In the supine and anaesthetised obese patient the increased weight acting on the diaphragm will reduce functional residual capacity and provoke significant basal atelectasis and hypoxaemia lasting well into the postoperative period.[12] These patients may also have cardiac ischaemia, diabetes, and hiatus hernia, are often difficult to intubate, and have poor venous access. Postoperatively they are at increased risk of venous thromboembolism (see above). They may occasionally require two operating tables. All in all, they pose a constellation of problems for the anaesthetist. Morbid obesity is a major risk factor at the time of surgery and needs to be recognised at an early stage.

Hepatic and renal systems

Poor hepatic function has several implications for the anaesthetist though these may only become apparent after biochemical screening. Prominent among these are coagulopathies which, if unrecognised, can result in unexpectedly heavy intraoperative bleeding or even spinal haematomata after regional block. Sensitivity to certain drugs, for example morphine, can result in prolonged sleepiness after anaesthesia because of reduced hepatic clearance. Ascites in hepatic cirrhosis may cause abdominal distension and splinting of the diaphragm with reduction in functional residual capacity and perioperative hypoxaemia. Intrapulmonary shunting may reduce oxygenation still further. Hypoglycaemia and sodium retention are additional metabolic abnormalities which need to be identified. Finally hepatitis poses a danger of needlestick injury to the nursing and medical staff.

Impairment of renal function may be acute (acute renal failure; ARF) or chronic (chronic renal failure; CRF). ARF can be the result of prerenal, renal or postrenal factors (Box 2.4). Reductions in renal function confer additional risks.[13] As well as impairment of drug excretion, the patient is unable to deal with the fluid loads administered in the perioperative period. In some patients a raised creatinine is only discovered during the preoperative work-up and necessitates review of the drug chart so that nephrotoxic drugs, for example diclofenac, can be excluded. For patients on renal support, it is important to identify the location of an arteriovenous shunt, check for anaemia and correct any fluid or electrolyte imbalance. These checks will have to be repeated in the postoperative period.

Endocrine system

Diabetes mellitus

The majority of patients (~80%) who suffer from diabetes are classed as type 2 diabetics (non-insulin dependent diabetes mellitus; NIDDM) and as such are treated with diet modification alone or with oral hypoglycaemic

Box 2.4 Causes of renal failure

Acute renal failure
Prerenal–hypovolaemia, hypotension, hypoxia
Renal–acute glomerulotubular necrosis, sepsis, nephrotoxins
Post renal–urinary tract obstruction

Chronic renal failure
Congenital–polycystic kidneys
Autoimmune disease–glomerulonephritis, rheumatoid arthritis, SLE
Infection–pyelonephritis
Urinary tract obstruction
Arterial disease–hypertension, diabetic arteriopathy

SLE, systemic lupus erythematosus

drugs. Most commonly these drugs are sulphonylureas (for example, glibenclamide or gliclazide) or biguanides (for example, metformin). The remainder of patients, generally a younger group with a tendency to develop ketoacidosis, will be type 1 insulin-dependent diabetics.

All diabetics are prone to microvascular damage and suffer end-organ disease, especially ischaemic heart disease, diabetic nephropathy, and neuropathies. For this reason, a thorough cardiac and renal assessment is essential. Autonomic neuropathy, which may impair vasomotor function and thus cause precipitous falls in blood pressure during anaesthesia, can be identified by a sustained fall in blood pressure on standing (orthostatic hypotension). In addition, diabetic retinopathy eventually affects 75% of all diabetic patients.

Once the timing of surgery is decided the objective in anaesthetic management of the diabetic is to provide the patient with good blood sugar control. Currently sliding scale insulin is the most popular perioperative regimen with concurrent administration of intravenous insulin and enough 10% glucose to satisfy metabolic demands. Regular measurements of blood sugar and urinary ketones in the perioperative period are important and represent good practice.

Thyroid disease

Evidence of thyroid over- or underactivity may be elucidated during the history or may be noticed during the clinical examination. Loss of weight associated with anxiety and tremor or intolerance to heat should lead to a physical examination of the neck. This should exclude swellings of a general or local type that may cause tracheal compression or deviation and thus interfere with airway management. Exophthalmos, apart from acting as a marker for thyroid malfunction, should be documented carefully so that special precautions to prevent corneal abrasions are taken during the anaesthetic.

Adrenal cortex

Disorders of adrenocortical function, though rare, may pose a significant threat to the patient during surgery and anaesthesia. Adrenocortical hyperfunction (Cushing's disease) is characterised by hypertension and muscle weakness and may co-exist with diabetes mellitus.

Patients with adrenocortical insufficiency (Addison's disease) feel generally unwell, weak with a history of anorexia, nausea and vomiting, abdominal pain, weight loss, postural hypotension, and skin pigmentation. Addison's commonly co-exists with diabetes mellitus, hypothyroidism, and hypoparathyroidism and may be caused by exogenous steroid administration.

Musculoskeletal system

Arthritis in its several forms can present the anaesthetist with many problems. Both rheumatoid and juvenile chronic arthritis cause systemic disorders including anaemia, renal, and cardiorespiratory disease. By far the worst difficulties seen in this group of patients are those affecting airway management. Arthritic temporomandibular joints may reduce mouth opening. Cervical spine immobility may be so severe that head extension is impossible. Laxity of the atlantoaxial joint ligaments and weakening of the odontoid peg can result in damage to the cervical cord during intubation. Preoperative airway assessment is thus critically important so that extra equipment such as fibreoptic endoscopes and staff with the necessary skills can be ready.

An associated problem in the arthritic patient is ulnar deviation of the hands with joint swelling. This can make venous access awkward and painful. Finally a drug history may reveal the use of immunosuppressive agents, non-steroidal antiinflammatory analgesics or penicillamine.

Special problems

The elderly

Elderly patients are an increasingly important section of the patient population. Old age is a risk factor during anaesthesia and surgery with an estimated 2–3 times the morbidity and mortality of lower age groups. Some authors suggest a general reduction in organ function of 1% per year once over the age of 30, though there is great variation between patients. Loss of functional reserve and a poor response to stress by the endocrine and cardiovascular systems are typical features of the elderly. Acting in concert with age-related diseases and their therapies, this combination of risk factors may present the anaesthetist with very significant difficulties.[14] In these patients a thorough drug history is not sufficient. Assessment of drug side effects must follow. Diuretic therapy may be associated with hypokalaemia, antiinflammatory agents with renal failure and steroids with a variety of side effects including electrolyte imbalance, adrenocortical suppression, and osteoporosis.

Sickle cell disease

All patients of Afro-Caribbean origins should be tested for sickle cell disease or trait. This group is prone to sickling during conditions of low oxygen levels, cold or acidosis, all of which may easily occur during anaesthesia. Tourniquets are a potential cause of sickling in the ischaemic limb and their use should be very carefully considered.

Trauma and burns

Patients with acute injuries constitute a difficult group. Inevitably, attention will be focused on the most pressing problem and a standard preoperative examination may be impossible. In these circumstances it is easy to get caught up in the general momentum of treatment and omit basic measures. However, it is important that the principles of care of the critically ill are remembered. Using the ABC sequence, airway management with cervical spine control is the first priority followed by correction of any respiratory disorders as well as circulation and haemorrhage control.

Patients with large burns may need early surgery. In addition to the standard preoperative examination and the exclusion of hypovolaemia, attention must be paid to the possibility of associated smoke inhalational injury. The presence of hoarseness, wheeze, a history of being burned in an enclosed space and evidence of soot particles in the nasopharynx are highly suggestive of smoke inhalation and are predictors of airway obstruction and postoperative respiratory failure.

Conclusion

A thorough preoperative history and examination before surgery will often identify patient risk factors. Most of these will be manageable. Taken in conjunction with appropriate laboratory and radiological investigations, a proper preoperative assessment will make a significant contribution to patient safety during the perioperative period.

1   Egan TD, Wong KC. Perioperative smoking cessation and anaesthesia. A review. *J Clin Anaesth* 1992; **4**: 63–72.
2   Alberti KGMM. Diabetes and surgery. *Anesthesiology* 1991; **74**: 209–11.
3   Ellis FR. The diagnosis of MH: its social implications. *Br J Anaesth* 1988; **60**: 251–2.
4   Lowe GDO, Greer IA, Cooke TG *et al*. Risk of and prophylaxis for venous thrombo-embolism in hospital patients. *BMJ* 1992; **305**: 567–73.
5   Dagnino J, Prys Roberts C. Strategy for patients with hypertensive heart disease. *Baillière's Clin Anaesthesiol* 1989; **3**: 261–89.
6   Howell SJ, Sear YM, Yeates D *et al*. Risk factors for cardiovascular death after elective surgery under general anaesthesia. *Br J Anaesth* 1998; **80**: 14–19.
7   Goldman L, Caldera DL, Nussbaum SR *et al*. Multifactorial index of cardiac risk in non-cardiac surgical procedures. *N Engl J Med* 1977; **97**: 845–50.
8   Goldman L. Cardiac risk in non cardiac surgery: an update. *Anesth Analg* 1995; **80**: 810–20.
9   Boyd O, Grounds RM, Bennett ED. A randomised clinical trial of the effect of a deliberate perioperative increase of oxygen delivery on mortality in high risk surgical patients. *JAMA* 1993; **270**: 2699–707.
10 Nunn JF, Milledge JS, Chen D *et al*. Respiratory criteria of fitness for surgery and anaesthesia. *Anaesthesia* 1988; **43**: 543–51.
11 Campbell NN. Respiratory tract infection and anaesthesia. *Anaesthesia* 1990; **45**: 561–2.
12 Hedenstierna G. Ventilation perfusion relationships during anaesthesia. *Thorax* 1995; **50**: 85–91.
13 Novis BK, Roizen MF, Aronsen S *et al*. Association of preoperative risk factors with post-operative renal failure. *Anesth Analg* 1994; **78**: 143–9.
14 Raja SN, Haythornthwaite JA. Anaesthetic management of the elderly. *Anesthesiology* 1999; **91**: 909–11.

3: Preoperative investigations

JOSEPH FOSS

Patient assessment in the perioperative period: the five "Ws"

Who?

Patients presenting for surgery will have a wide variation in their prior contact with the medical community. At one extreme is the patient who has self-referred to a surgeon for a specific problem, say a painful knee, and aside from the surgical evaluation very little medical history is available. This may be the case even in the presence of several underlying medical conditions. Alternatively, the patient may be under the regular care of a general physician (GP), who has identified a potential problem and referred the patient to a surgeon. The surgeon or internist may have already requested the evaluation of other consultant specialists such as a cardiologist.

In the former situation, the anaesthesiologist may have to take the initiative in evaluating the medical status of the patient. This will include the initial examination, the selection of tests and ultimately may involve referral of the patient to a GP for initiation of therapy for preexisting medical conditions. In the latter case, a complete medical history with extensive data about the patient will already be available. In both of these situations, the patient will still need further assessment by an anaesthesiologist prior to surgery. There are a variety of points on which the anaesthesiologist has the most expertise.

The anaesthesiologist will be managing the patient's medical condition during the stress of surgery. These stresses may far surpass any that the patient experiences on a day-to-day basis living at home. The anaesthesiologist will be managing the patient under the influence of the anaesthetic drugs. These drugs are unique to the perioperative period in most cases and have a wide range of haemodynamic effects and drug interactions. Anaesthesia frequently involves the obtunding of airway reflexes and the requirement for airway management and mechanical ventilation. Even relatively "healthy" patients may have their anaesthetic plans altered based on the preoperative evaluation.[1] Assessment and optimisation of any under-lying medical conditions, in the light of the planned anaesthetic, is the foundation for a safe perioperative experience for the patient. See Chapters 4 and 6.

When?

The testing rationale (below) would suggest that if investigations are being done with an view to optimising the patient's condition preoperatively the results of those tests must be available and reviewed in time to allow for intervention should it be required. Patients who arrive for surgery and are evaluated immediately preoperatively are a source of delays and cancellations in the operating rooms. A preoperative visit 5–7 working days prior to the scheduled surgery allows time to review results of laboratory investigations and to initiate therapy for problems. This can decrease day-of-surgery delays or cancellations.[2] Such a visit may be planned to coincide with a scheduled visit to the surgeon or handled as a scheduled "walk-in", minimising the inconvenience to the patient.

Why?

There is a significant body of data that demonstrates that preoperative patient conditions are potential indicators of perioperative morbidity.[3-6] Fowkes and colleagues examined seven major preoperative conditions, adjusted them for the preoperative clinical assessment of the patient's condition and found that mortality was lower if a given condition was present in the patient in better condition.[7] The presence of cardiac failure, for example, increased mortality to 5.3% from a baseline of 0.2% in patients in good condition, but this was significantly lower than the 20.8% mortality seen for failure patients in poor condition. The extension of these observations is that optimising these conditions and planning operative management for them will minimise such morbidity. The approach to such an evaluation, however, should be focused.

Routine testing, i.e. testing performed on all patients regardless of their medical condition or the need for the information obtained, has no place in current medical practice. Tests may be done in large populations for screening purposes but generally, screening is inappropriate without an explicit goal for care of the patient presenting for surgery.

Testing should be performed to evaluate the patient's medical condition and physiology so that, when possible, their condition can be optimised preoperatively and to allow for planning of the management of the anaesthetic and course of surgery by the anaesthesiologist. The tests may affect the intensity of planned monitoring, the selection of anaesthetic agents, and postoperative disposition and care plan.

What?

This is the crux of the chapter. The goal of preoperative testing should be optimal utilisation (not minimal testing, which tends to eliminate even useful tests). The decision on which tests are used must be based on a testing rationale, and knowledge of the information provided by the test in the setting of that rationale. We will proceed with a review of the principles of testing, for the reader must understand how to evaluate a test's performance in planning test utilisation.

Impact of surgical severity on preoperative assessment
A decade ago no distinction would be made for patients presenting for preoperative assessment related to the type of surgery. Advances in surgical techniques and the availability of new anaesthetic techniques for rapid emergence have enabled us to provide a surgical experience with minimal impact on the patient. This in turn is leading to a reexamination of how we prepare patients for surgery. Pasternak has suggested that we may be able to triage patients to the type of preoperative evaluation they are given.[8] Based on a patient's ASA classification of Physical Status and the potential for the anticipated surgery to produce stress and haemodynamic changes, we could potentially triage patients into one of three categories: patients who must be seen in a preoperative clinic; patients for whom preadmission assessment is advisable; and those for whom preoperative assessment can be deferred until the morning of the procedure (Table 3.1). We are exploring this approach at our institution.

Table 3.1 Physical status and surgical severity in determining the need for preadmission anaesthetic assessment

	Surgical severity		
ASA PS	Minimally invasive (e.g. cataract, diagnostic arthroscopy)	Moderately invasive (e.g. carotid endarterectomy, cholecystectomy)	Highly invasive (e.g. total hip replacement, aortic surgery)
I	Optional	Recommended	Required
II	Optional	Recommended	Required
III	Recommended	Recommended	Required
IV	Required	Required	Required

The preoperative anaesthetic assessment may be done in a formal setting such as a clinic with an anaesthesiologist, screened by automated means or by support staff or in the immediate preoperative period. This triage can be based on the patient's general health and the anticipated severity of the surgery. A similar scoring system may be used in determining the level of ancillary testing used in the clinic. There are currently no prospective trials of such a triage system and each institution may have a different tolerance for which type of patient may have a minimal evaluation prior to the day of surgery.

ASA PS, American Society of Anesthesiologists Physical Status

37

Where?

Historically every patient coming for surgery was admitted to the hospital at least the night before his or her planned procedure. This provided an opportunity for the anaesthesiologist to meet and examine the patient, make an assessment, and an anaesthetic plan. The hospital setting offered some capability for obtaining additional information and tests should they be required, but there were limits to what could be accomplished overnight. Recent trends in surgery have altered this dynamic.

Outpatient surgery and same-day admission for surgery has become the norm, accounting for more than 50% of the surgical volume in many institutions. In our facility, this has extended to even the major cases such as coronary artery bypass and lung resections. During the transition to this new system many anaesthesiologists have been faced with meeting the majority of their patients in a preoperative holding area on the day of surgery. Additionally, many of these patients are complex and have reams of data with them (or worse, reams of data in medical records which are unavailable).

Anaesthesiologists and surgical facilities are now actively exploring alternatives to this situation. A dedicated preoperative clinic gives the opportunity for a careful history and examination, which (along with other benefits such as the patient interaction in a less pressured environment) can allow for optimal use of investigations. If the resources for such a clinic are not available, screening programmes utilising paper questionnaires, telephone interviews or electronically administered health screens can provide a basis for triage and selective in-depth evaluation of patients (Table 3.1). This analogy could be extended to the nature of ancillary preoperative testing which is done. For example, no testing at all may be needed in the patient presenting for a minimally invasive procedure. In a recent, prospective randomised study of morbidity and mortality in 19 577 patients for cataract surgery, Schein and colleagues concluded that routine tests, which were not otherwise indicated by the patient's health, provided no benefit.[9] The underlying assumptions of this approach, however, are that patients are seen by some health-care provider preoperatively and that the provider can make a reliable estimate of both the patient's health status and the invasiveness of the upcoming surgery.

Principles of testing

Developing a testing rationale

Testing should be performed to evaluate the patient's medical condition and physiology so that, when possible, their condition can be optimised preoperatively and to allow for planning of the management of the anaesthetic and course of surgery by the anaesthesiologist. The tests may affect the intensity of planned monitoring, the selection of anaesthetic agents, and postoperative disposition and care plan.

Evaluating test performance

Test performance, at its most basic definition, is the ability to provide valuable data and to do so with fewer negative effects than positive effects at a reasonable cost. The definition of performance for any test is in fact a very dynamic process. It relates to the test, the population being examined, and the value of the data to the clinician in a given circumstance.

Sensitivity

Sensitivity is the ability of a test to identify the presence of disease. Let us examine a commonly discussed (but imaginary) disease: having a cracked pot. Having a cracked pot is defined as having a serum porcelain level outside the normal range of 0.5–4.95 International Units. If having a cracked pot has a true prevalence of 10% (i.e. 100 of 1000 subjects from the entire population tested have cracked pots) and the test identifies 95 of those 100 positively, then its sensitivity is 95%. The test will also have missed five patients with disease, the false negatives.

Sensitivity is in fact difficult to apply to many of the tests ordered preoperatively. Many tests report not the presence of disease but rather the abnormality of a value defined as a number at either end of a range of normal values (for example, a hypothetical test of serum hyperporcelainaemia, indicative of the presence of a "cracked pot"). In that case, the test has a fixed sensitivity (95% in the case of abnormal being defined as 2 standard deviations away from the mean), but the actual value does not designate any specific disease, just those subjects who stray from the normal population. On the other hand, if the disease is defined by being more than the preselected difference from the mean, sensitivity will approach 100%. Why will it not be 100%? If the test were repeated on the same individual sample, there is a small chance that it would return a normal value (related to the precision of the test), but most modern automated tests have very high precision.

Specificity

Specificity is the ability of a test to identify the absence of disease in health. In other words, a good test will not label healthy patients as being abnormal. Following our previous example, it is unlikely that the test would identify exactly 95 subjects as having cracked pots and that they would all be truly abnormal. If the test has a specificity of 98%, it will identify 98% of the 900 healthy patients as disease free or normal. The test will also define 2% of the 900, or 18 patients, as false positive for having cracked pots. Therefore the test will have labelled 95+18=113 patients as having cracked pots.

39

Specificity and sensitivity are characteristics of the test being done. They are, in the absence of interfering physiological factors that might change the performance of the test, related to the test alone and not the population or individual in whom we are doing the test. An important caveat is that the test must have been validated on a population that provides a valid comparison group to the target population. An individual test may also have different sensitivity and specificity for different endpoints. The 12-lead electrocardiogram is both highly sensitive and specific for rhythm abnormalities but has much poorer sensitivity and specificity for the presence of ischaemic disease.

What is more important, sensitivity or specificity? For many tests, these characteristics are at odds. You can define abnormal levels to enhance sensitivity at the cost of specificity, or vice versa. This is where the testing rationale again comes into play. Why are you doing the test? If you are screening large populations for a common disease with serious consequences which you do not want to miss (such as hyperbilirubinaemia at birth), you will emphasise sensitivity. If the consequences of a positive test have significant treatment, economic or social consequences (such as HIV testing) you will put a higher value on specificity, making sure that you are not inadvertently treating large numbers of healthy people. That brings us to the combination of testing characteristics with population characteristics.

Prior predictive value
In our example, if one does no testing, there is a 1 in 10 chance that any person coming to the operating room has a cracked pot. If having a cracked pot has consequences for the anaesthetic plan, say dysphoria after morphine, one might obtain a serum porcelain level preoperatively to help decide if morphine can be used as part of the anaesthetic. Now there are two populations. If the test result is negative (n=1000 −113 or 887), the probability that my patient has a cracked pot is only 0.6% (five false negatives in 887 patients labelled negative) and the anaesthesiologist can proceed without altering the plan. If the test is positive, 95 of those 113 patients, or 84%, will have the condition and the anaesthesiologist will not use morphine.

Conditions of importance to the anaesthesiologist are rarely as common as 10% in the unselected population. If having a cracked pot had the same incidence of malignant hyperthermia in the US (for example, 1:50 000) and the test had the same sensitivity of 95% and specificity of 98%, the clinical value of the information is markedly different. The odds of a patient with a negative test having MH goes from very small (0.00002) to very, very small (0.000001) but the odds of a patient with a positive test having MH remain at very small (0.001). It is difficult to rationalise a change in practice based on the presence of a positive test. Either we need a better test or we need to improve the odds that the patient has the disease in the first place. Simply eliciting a positive history from the patient of a first-degree relative with a history of MH symptoms during an anaesthetic puts the patient in a population

40

where 1:1000 will have MH. Now the test has a markedly improved predictive value.

Informatics

Test selection relies on a detailed understanding of the performance of individual tests in selected populations. New tests and refinements to guidelines for testing are produced regularly. The clinician faced with making an informed test selection would ideally take the time to do a thorough review of systems (encompassing up to 100 items) and then integrate this with the data on available tests. In reality, most of us face limitations in our time, patience, and skill which result in hitting the high points, focusing on those areas where our instincts might lead us, and perhaps ordering some excess tests to cover potential gaps in our knowledge. An alternative is to develop tools to assist in test selection.

Patient questionnaires and checklists exist which are often more extensive than oral review of systems. These may be coupled with algorithms that recommend tests. These systems must provide a linear set of questions or they quickly become unwieldy (if "yes" go to question 35, otherwise skip to question 42….). This limits their ability to go into depth in areas where a problem is identified. Additionally, the presentation of the information is neither logical nor condensed for the reviewer.

Computer systems are designed for such repetitive, branched logic tasks. The data may be collected in a series of questions logical to the patient, with varying depth and series based on patient characteristics, and then analysed and organised for optimal use by the clinician. A limitation of this process has been the access to such computer-based systems.

HealthQuiz® is one such system.* It selects approximately 100 questions from a set of 167 based on patient characteristics and previous question answers. The data are organised into a systematic report of pertinent positive and negatives and recommendations as to appropriate laboratory testing are made. The system is Internet based (www.healthquiz.com) and can be accessed by any computer with a Web browser and recently has been adapted to accept input from the patient over a touch-tone phone. The other advantages of such a system include patient convenience, a central repository for information, a continuously updated set of questions and guidelines, and the redirecting of physician time from asking routine questions to dealing with issues which have already been identified.

---

* HealthQuiz has been developed at the University of Chicago and funds derived from its use return to its licensee, University Community Health Care Inc. The University of Chicago, the Department of Anesthesia and Critical Care and Johns Hopkins University of Baltimore may benefit from commercialisation of this technology and the applications described herein.

Testing follies

More tests are better

It is a commonly held belief that having more data is always better and that once you have decided to obtain any tests, you might as well get them all. The only negative aspect of testing for the patient in this scenario is the initial venepuncture. There are several direct and indirect consequences of excess testing, however. As we have already shown, no test performs perfectly. A certain number of patients who are normal will be misidentified as abnormal by any test and if the test is not indicated, the proportion of false positives may actually rise. Abnormal tests which are identified frequently lead to additional testing, from repeating the same test to potentially significantly more invasive procedures. Even if the additional tests are normal, they add little clinical value. Every test has a dollar cost associated with it. Even if a specific test cost is trivial in the setting of an individual surgery, excess preoperative testing in the United States has been estimated to consume 30 billion $US annually. These funds are no longer available for providing care, which may have improved patient health. As well as consuming funds, unindicated tests, even if normal, must consume some time and energy in their review, distracting the physician from tasks which may be of more benefit to the patient.

Defensive testing

Physicians express concern that they will be held liable if there is a bad outcome from surgery that might have been identified by obtaining a test preoperatively (many of our surgeons insist on routine prothrombin (PT) to partial thromboplastin time (PTT) for tonsillectomies). This argument stands neither to reason nor to examination of practice. If a test is not indicated prior to surgery by history or examination and this is documented, there will be no grounds for practising outside the standard of care, which is required to demonstrate malpractice. It has also been shown that physicians may expose themselves to a new risk. Tests ordered without a clear indication are frequently not reviewed and if they produce abnormal test values, they are often not noted or the results are disregarded. This ignorance or disregard for a documented abnormality clearly could be construed as practice below the standard of care.

Ethics of investigations

We generally think of informed consent as it is applied to major procedures, but the principles behind such consent apply to the anaesthesia perioperative assessment. The patient has the right to know what examinations and tests we are going to perform, the potential benefits and risks involved, the right to decline those investigations, and what the consequences of such a decision would be (see also Chapter 7). We rarely engage in a formal discussion of these issues over something as straightforward as a full blood count, but I would challenge the physician ordering such a test to be able to respond to a patient should all those questions arise. Many "routine" tests would fail a rigorous examination of these points (for example, even the transient pain and small risk of a bruise over the site of venepuncture outweighs the value of obtaining the sample when not having the sample would have no effect on the clinical care of the patient). Further, if the tests are being obtained for non-clinical reasons (medicolegal, financial, etc.) the possibility of violating the rights of the patient increases.

Some tests have significant questions associated with their performance. These tend to be tests where the discovery of a positive finding has repercussions beyond the surgery itself. Two such tests are for human immuno-deficiency virus (HIV) and pregnancy.

Testing for pregnancy in women of childbearing potential has been examined in several settings. The two primary concerns are fetal demise and fetal malformations. The teratogenic effects of the majority of anaesthetic agents currently in use appear to be low. The rate of fetal loss during anaesthesia and surgery is somewhat more significant but it is difficult to separate the effects of the anaesthetics from the effects of surgical stress. In the situation where a woman knows she may be pregnant or is attempting to become pregnant, it is clear that testing should be done so that she can weigh the potential risks to the pregnancy against the benefits of the planned surgery. In women who deny that they are possibly pregnant the rate of positive pregnancy is 0.3–0.49%.[10,11] In both this group and those who are unsure of their status but who are not actively seeking a pregnancy, we believe a brief discussion of the risks should be made and pregnancy testing done with the specific consent of the woman. Specific plans should be available in the event that an unplanned pregnancy is discovered in terms of providing support and counselling for the patient.

HIV is treated by many health-care professionals not only as an issue with prolonged impact on the patient, but one with public health implications and potentially increased risk to the health-care practitioner. In many areas HIV testing cannot be done without the specific written consent of the patient and the results are handled with a higher degree of confidentiality than the rest of the medical record. HIV screening in a general population without risk factors has a very low yield of true positives and a high rate of false positives, unless redundant testing is performed, with the attendant anxiety until the test can be repeated and confirmed or denied.[12] Testing in patients with known risk factors, which will vary widely in prevalence from region to region, performs more favourably.

The next question is: how does the knowledge that a patient is HIV positive affect our care of the patient? We should use universal precautions against infections for all of our patients, as there are many diseases more common, more easily transmitted and as fatal as HIV in our patient populations (for example, hepatitis B and C). Asymptomatic patients with HIV who are not on drug therapy (many of the drugs for HIV treatment have multiple drug–drug interactions) do not present any special challenges for the anaesthesiologist. Again, if the patient has risk factors but no indications of HIV infection, a discussion with the patient about the risk and benefits of early detection of the disease and its impact on the surgery and anaesthesia is in order and the patient should be allowed to decide if they want the test done. Indeed, asking the patient if they want a test for HIV may be one of the easiest ways to allow patients to self-identify themselves as being in a risk group without getting into sensitive lifestyle discussions.

Assessment of the cardiovascular system

The principal concerns for the cardiovascular system include congestive heart failure (CHF), ischaemic disease, valvular disease, hypertension, cardiomyopathies, rhythm abnormalities, and signs of atherosclerosis.[13] A careful history will elicit risk factors, which can direct subsequent testing. These tests should provide data to quantify the current disease state and to direct preoperative interventions and intraoperative management. Guidelines for the perioperative evaluation of cardiac risk in patients for non-cardiac surgery have been developed (and are available on the Web at www.acc.org/clincal/guidelines).[14]

Vascular disease

Vascular disease can represent both a marker of underlying problems as well as a significant problem in and of itself. The aetiology of vascular disease will often be apparent in the history and a variety of findings on physical examination can assist in determining the severity of the disease.

A family history of morbidity and mortality related to vascular diseases, such as stroke and myocardial infarction, increases the risk for any patient that they may be susceptible to the same conditions. Hypercholesterolaemia has both hereditary and lifestyle components that may be sought. Diabetes, and how the patient has managed their disease, will be a strong indicator of the potential for vascular problems.

A personal history of previous transient ischaemic attacks, stroke, carotid endarterectomy, myocardial ischaemia or revascularisation and peripheral revascularisation procedures are of course diagnostic. More importantly, the presence of disease in any one area then mandates a more extensive examination of the other systems to document the extent of the disease.

Physical findings begin with simple observational items such evidence of facial droop or weakness consistent with prior stroke or the presence of previous amputations due to vascular disease. Vascular insufficiency will produce characteristic changes of skin in the extremities. Examination should be made of the peripheral and carotid pulses for quality, amplitude, and bruits.

Positive findings are going to direct the nature of any additional work-up. The presence of peripheral vascular disease, even in the absence of cardiac ischaemic symptomatology, is a strong indicator for the need to consider additional examinations of the heart. The serum lipid profile can assess the presence of hypercholesterolaemia or the success of control if the patient has been started on cholesterol-lowering drugs. There has been recent interest in markers of the general inflammatory state of the body, such as C-reactive protein, as indicators of the degree of potential vascular susceptibility to plaque formation, rupture or thrombosis.[15–17] The value of the indicators in the acute perioperative period has not been examined but they have some predictive value in both longitudinal studies of cardiovascular disease and the setting of acute myocardial infarction.

Cardiac rhythm

12-lead electrocardiogram (ECG)
A history encompassing ischaemic risk factors, palpitations, syncope in combination with palpation of pulses and auscultation of the chest will provide the rationale for obtaining a 12-lead ECG in most cases. Abnormalities on ECG are relatively common and increase with age to 10% of the population at 40 and 25% of the population at 60, often prompting "age triggers" in obtaining ECGs. In asymptomatic patients over the age of 60 who have been shown to have no perioperatively significant symptoms, only two of 163 patients older than 60 had important abnormalities. In asymptomatic patients under age 40 only 0.6% have been shown to have significant abnormalities.[18]

The presence of a normal ECG within the previous two years does not decrease the likelihood of new abnormalities on a repeat ECG[19, 20] but a history of a previously abnormal ECG does indicate a 25–40% increased probability of there being new ECG abnormalities. This would suggest that, if indicated, a new ECG should be obtained if the previous ECG is more than two months old, whether the previous ECG was normal or abnormal.

Cardiac performance

Congestive heart failure is a significant risk factor for perioperative morbidity.[5, 21] The difficulty of managing an anaesthetic in a patient with an ejection fraction of less than 30% is readily appreciated. The more difficult patient is one who has marginal function (ejection fraction of 30–45%) who may appear to be functionally capable of tolerating an anaesthetic but who in fact may also be at increased risk.

45

The history of symptoms consistent with congestive failure, along with an assessment of the maximum amount of effort the patient can exert, will form the basis for additional examinations. The presence of cardiomegaly, rales, and murmurs on exam along with peripheral oedema should be noted.

Echocardiography (ECHO)

The cardiac echo study has become a cornerstone of cardiac evaluation. It is non-invasive, or in the case of the transoesophageal procedure moderately invasive, but usually well tolerated. It provides both structural and functional information about the heart muscle and valves and the addition of stress echocardiography has increased the sensitivity and specificity of the technique for ischaemia.[22,23]

It is a moderately expensive test that is typically available as an outpatient procedure, frequently with little delay. It requires sophisticated equipment, especially for advanced flow and multiplanar studies of the valves. A close working relationship with an experienced team for obtaining and interpreting the studies will significantly improve its value to the anaesthesiologist.

Anaesthesiologists, in turn, will obtain the most value if they can be specific about the information required from the study. The presence of decreased myocardial performance may indicate the need for not only increased intraoperative monitoring of volume, but careful attention on postoperative days 2 and 3 as fluids from the periphery are mobilised back into the central circulation.

Cardiac ischaemia

Patients will fall into three broad categories easily recognised by the clinician:

- active and fit patients with few cardiac risk factors
- patients with documented cardiac ischaemic disease
- patients with cardiac risk factors but no history or current symptoms of disease in whom the risk of intraoperative ischaemia is unclear.

The trend for the first group is to increasingly minimise any evaluation which might be done, even in the older patient. The second group will frequently have already had an extensive evaluation of their disease and possibly have had some form of revascularisation. Again, the trend for additional evaluation if there have been no interval changes in the patient's symptoms would be to not repeat studies such as a stress test done within the last two years. Changes in symptoms or functional status suggestive of progression of the disease warrant a return visit to the patient's primary care physician for an update of their condition and possible adjustment of their care programme.

The third group has been the focus of extensive study, discussion, and development of a variety of algorithms to attempt to optimise the evaluation and therapy of these patients. The American College of Cardiology and American Heart Association, with input from the anaesthesia community, produced a set of guidelines on the evaluation of the patient with cardiac disease for non-cardiac surgery that included cost–benefit analysis of the various options.[14] Although they have been widely disseminated, it is our impression that there is still significant variability in the application of these guidelines. Further, technology continues to advance with improved diagnostic and therapeutic options that have not been incorporated yet.

12-lead electrocardiogram

The resting ECG has low sensitivity and specificity as a screening tool for the presence of myocardial ischaemia or the risk of developing worsening ischaemia during the operation. The presence of Q waves, however, is part of the algorithm for proceeding with additional evaluation (Box 3.1). It is also one of the primary intraoperative monitors used for ischaemia and the baseline ECG can be used to assess the presence of abnormalities such as bundle branch block which will decrease its usefulness and possibly indicate the need for additional monitors as well as providing a comparator for intraoperative changes.

Box 3.1 Referring patients undergoing non-cardiac surgery for additional evaluation of cardiovascular risk

Indicators for ECG	Indicators for additional evaluation
Chest pain	Myocardial infarction
Angina	Recurrent angina
Congestive heart failure	Congestive heart failure
Hypertension	Diabetes on treatment
Diabetes	Q waves on ECG
Dysrhythmia	
Dyspnoea	
Myocardial infarction	
Age >39 male, >49 female	
Smoking history	
Vascular disease	
Intrathoracic tumour	
NONE of above – proceed with non-cardiac surgery	NONE of above – proceed with non-cardiac surgery
ANY of above – obtain ECG	1–2 of above – non-invasive evaluation (Table 3.2)
	3 or more of above – preoperative cardiac catheterisation

Non-invasive stress tests and invasive assessment

Box 3.1 and Table 3.2 summarise the approach to evaluating the cardiac risk for the patient presenting for non-cardiac surgery. This is a very dynamic area and it is likely that new studies such as the fast CT evaluation and new therapies such as stenting will lead to rapid evolution of the algorithm. There are also institution-specific differences in capabilities that may dictate the preferred types of evaluation.

Table 3.2 Additional evaluation of cardiac risk in the patient for non-cardiac surgery

Non-invasive test	Result	Follow-up	Action
Holter and ST-segment monitoring for 24 hours	(-) < 1h ischaemia		Proceed
	(+) > 1h ischaemia	Catheterisation	
		Surgery/PTCA/stent	Proceed
		Non-correctable	Increase intra- and postop monitoring
Dipyridamole echocardiography	(-)Fixed wall motion abnormalities		Increase intra- and postop monitoring
	(+)Dynamic wall motion abnormalities	Catheterisation	
		Surgery/PTCA/stent	Proceed
		Non-correctable	Increase intra- and postop monitoring
Stress (exercise or pharmacological) thallium testing	(-)Fixed perfusion defects		Increase intra- and postop monitoring
	(+)Dynamic perfusion defects	Catheterisation	
		Surgery/PTCA/stent	Proceed
		Non-correctable	Increase intra- and postop monitoring

The patient should be referred for additional non-invasive testing based on criteria in Box 3.1. The cardiologist will select the mode of testing with which the institution has the most expertise. Increased monitoring implies invasive monitors and three days of intensive care postoperatively.

PTCA, percutaneous transluminal coronary angioplasty

Working with consultants

Anaesthesiologists have constantly decried the typical note from a consultant which summarises the patient's condition and then closes: "*Avoid hypoxia and hypotension. Patient cleared for anaesthesia*". Consultations with specialists can be an important part of the anaesthesia perioperative assessment but they can also represent a significant cost to the system and inconvenience to the patient if they have to make additional arrangements for another clinic visit. Furthermore, they frequently result in additional testing which has both associated risks and costs. The anaesthesiologist must take responsibility to ensure that the information they seek is obtained from the consultant.

In our clinic we have instituted a system where both the indication for the consultation and the desired information is specified (Box 3.2). This is done by electronically generating a letter in our clinic, but could be replicated with a check-off form. It will be noted that we do not specify how the consultant should evaluate a given condition (for example, requesting a stress thallium test); rather we request that the consultant apply their expertise in addressing the clinical problem. This system allows us to assess both the appropriateness of the request by the anaesthesiologist as well as the quality of the response with regard to providing specific data for the perioperative management of the patient.

We discourage our surgeons from obtaining routine preoperative assessments by consultants prior to the anaesthesia perioperative assessment, as the need for such an evaluation and the information required may not be well defined. That is not to say that we discourage participation in preoperative preparation by the patient's regular internist or cardiologist. A letter or recent notes from office visits can be invaluable as an adjunct to understanding the patient's disease state. They should obtain new studies that are appropriate in the overall context of the patient's disease. What we wish to avoid is having them obtain a new study "... *in case anaesthesia wants it*".

Box 3.2 Indications and requested information for consultants

---

Indications
The patient has:
- poorly controlled hypertension
- poorly controlled angina
- poorly controlled asthma
- poorly controlled COPD
- new ECG changes and CAD risk factors
- multiple underevaluated cardiac risk factors
- history of cardiac ischaemia with no recent assessment
- history of cardiac failure with no recent assessment
- history of pulmonary failure with no recent assessment
- history of asthma with no recent assessment

Information requested
Recent clinic note
Recent laboratory tests (within eight weeks) and last ECG (any)
Evaluate:
- hypertension and initiate treatment
- risk for perioperative ischaemia
- cardiac ischaemia and optimise treatment
- patient's baseline cardiac function
- patient's cardiac function and optimise treatment
- patient's baseline pulmonary function
- pulmonary function and optimise treatment
Reevaluate:
- current medical status and treatments

Assessment of the pulmonary system

A history of chronic obstructive pulmonary disease, orthopnoea, and dyspnoea on mild exertion or at rest is indicative of underlying pulmonary disease. Cardiovascular disease and a history of malignancy may also indicate the need for evaluation of the pulmonary system.

Pulmonary x ray

If the history is positive, obtain a chest radiograph (CXR) if none has been done within the last year. Tape and colleagues[24] look at the practice of routine CXR in 341 patients for vascular surgery. While an abnormal CXR was associated with a higher rate of complications, all the beneficial effects attributed to the CXR accrued in patients with clinical evidence of disease. Also, six patients faced potentially clinically detrimental false-positive or false-negative diagnosis due to the CXR. Additional indications include a pulmonary infection with a productive cough, patients at risk for exposure to tuberculosis or other chest disease (travel or occupation) or any interval change in symptoms or invasive thoracic procedures. The CXR may also be a valuable adjunct in assessing the airway and trachea in patients with mediastinal lesions or other risk factors (as may be any CT that has frequently been obtained in anticipation of the surgery).

Pulmonary function tests (PFTs)

If the reversibility of bronchospasm needs to be determined, PFTs with bronchodilators are indicated. The presence of severe disease may warrant obtaining baseline function for comparison when trying to determine the patient's readiness for extubation postoperatively. Finally, if the patient is scheduled for lung resection, maximum breathing capacity, carbon monoxide diffusing capacity, and maximum mid-expiratory flow rate should be obtained.

Assessment of haematology and coagulation

Haemoglobin, haematocrit, and white blood cell count

The only abnormality of circulating blood cells that has been shown to impact on perioperative morbidity is uncontrolled polycythaemia.[25] Normovolaemic anaemia has not been demonstrated to be a risk factor and patients undergoing anaesthesia and minor surgery with haemoglobin levels above 8 g/dl have not been seen to be at increased risk.[26,27] There are no significant data to suggest that white cell abnormalities impact on surgical outcome. Thus, we must arbitrarily set relatively liberal preoperative values which may be tolerated (haematocrit 29–57% for men, 27–54% for women, white blood count [WBC] 2400–16 000/mm³). The importance of abnormalities outside these ranges lies more in the identification of the source of the abnormality as it may otherwise impact on the patient's health.

Asymptomatic patients do not generally fall outside these ranges and testing for minor surgery is not indicated. Patients undergoing more significant procedures who are female or men over the age of 40 should have a haematocrit or haemoglobin done. If blood loss in excess of 2 units/70 kg is anticipated a preoperative type and screen may be done. A history of smoking, anticoagulant use, malignancy or renal disease is also an indication for a haemoglobin or haematocrit.

Obtaining a WBC is rarely indicated preoperatively. If the patient has a malignancy or has recently undergone chemotherapy or has signs and symptoms of an acute infectious process, the WBC should be performed. An automated or manual differential is usually only needed in situations where the aetiology of the elevated WBC count is unclear.

Platelets and coagulation factors

Patients who are active and asymptomatic are unlikely to have disorders of the coagulation system that will affect their surgery. A history enquiring about easy bruising (for example, the patient gets bruises and does not know where they came from), unusual bleeding of the gums or from cuts and the use of drugs which affect the coagulation system should guide testing. Co-existing conditions of renal disease, hepatic disease, malnutrition, systemic lupus erythematosus, and major trauma are also indications for testing.

The platelet count can vary significantly and still be acceptable for surgery. This test does not evaluate platelet function. The bleeding time is frequently used but when it is not markedly prolonged it does not correlate well with the effects of antiplatelet drugs such as aspirin on the risk of bleeding with nerve blocks or intraoperative blood loss.[28]

The prothrombin time (PT) and activated partial thromboplastin time (aPTT) represent the specific intrinsic and extrinsic pathways of coagulation. In the absence of a history of clinical bleeding, a family or personal history of genetic disorders of the pathways or the use of anticoagulants, the likelihood of a true positive test is low.[29, 30]

Assessment of serum biochemistry

One of the first considerations for evaluation of serum chemistry is that the studies are still routinely done as "panels". Doing a panel of 20 tests, each based on a population norm where values more than 2 standard deviations away from the mean are flagged, has a 64% chance of producing at least one test that would be abnormal, though the patient has no clinical disease.

Thus, where indicated, specific tests should be done and pursuit of unexpected abnormalities with no clinical correlation should be avoided. In general, for asymptomatic patients less than 65 years of age, no testing in this area is indicated.

Renal function

The kidneys eliminate many drugs and their metabolites. They are involved in a variety of diseases as well as being sensitive to many drugs. Blood urea nitrogen and serum creatinine are primary indicators of renal function and should be obtained in the presence of a history of renal disease or diabetes, liver disease, morbid obesity, and steroid or diuretic use.

Hepatic function

The liver is both an important organ in the metabolism of many of our anaesthetics and a potential target for toxicity. As noted above, it also plays an important synthetic role in the coagulation system. The presence of known liver disease, a history of jaundice, exposure to hepatitis, alcohol abuse, unexplained weight loss, unusual changes in bowel habits or stool colour or gastrointestinal bleeding are indications for obtaining liver function tests. A variety of drugs such as cholesterol-lowering agents require monitoring of liver functions and these should have been done within the schedule suggested by the manufacturer.[31]

Metabolic, electrolyte, and endocrine abnormalities

Glucose levels should be evaluated in the presence of diabetes or symptoms suggestive of diabetes such as nocturia or morbid obesity. Central nervous system disease or planned surgery on the central nervous system are also indications for a serum glucose in view of the sensitivity of the brain under ischaemia to hyperglycaemia. The use of hypoglycaemic agents and steroids will also affect glucose levels.

Thyroid dysfunction can be sought by characteristic changes of under- or overproduction. Significant disease should produce a clear history of heat or cold intolerance, changes in weight, and constitutional symptoms.

Adrenal disease is uncommon but an undiagnosed phaeochromocytoma can be fatal under anaesthesia. Again, constitutional symptoms of hyperactivity such as episodic sweating or flushing without exercise must be sought and referral for testing and therapy made if they are identified.

The most frequent cause of electrolyte abnormalities will be iatrogenic. The use of drugs such as diuretics and steroids is associated with a variety of abnormal findings. The acute or chronic nature of changes is often important, as patients will tolerate a gradual drift towards extremes better than a sudden change. This is another example where the cure may be worse than the disease. Identification of asymptomatic hypokalaemia has not been associated with adverse perioperative outcomes.[32,33] Acute replenishment of potassium to achieve normal levels, however, has led to morbidity.[34,35]

Under-ordering of tests

The last two decades have seen an extensive reexamination of preoperative evaluation based both on balancing the risks and benefits of testing and, more recently, on minimising expenditures for such evaluation. This has led, unfortunately, to the potential for under-ordering tests. Macario and colleagues evaluated these changes and found that while unindicated testing had been significantly reduced in institutions with an awareness of the issue, indicated testing had decreased almost 1.5 times as fast.[36] This is unacceptable as it may obviously also lead to delays on the day of surgery or adverse patient outcomes. It is particularly troubling when this under-ordering is driven by shortsighted cost-cutting measures.

Optimising test utilisation

Roizen has put forward the notion of the optimum curve for preoperative evaluation (Fig. 3.1).[37] Providers must change their perspective from one of

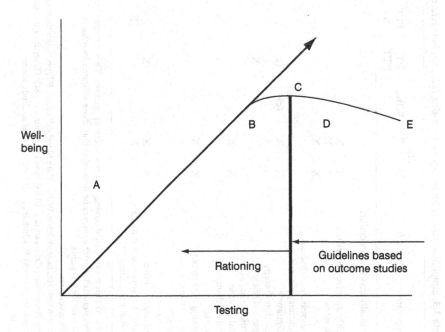

Figure 3.1 Optimisation of preoperative testing.

Table 3.3 Simplified strategy for preoperative testing (adapted from reference [38])

Preoperative condition (a)	Hb		WBC	PT/ PTT	PLT/ BT	ELECT	Cr/ BUN	GLU	SGOT/ ALK P	CXR	ECG	ALB	T/S
	M	F											
Minimally invasive procedure (b)													
Highly invasive procedure	X	X					X	X			X	X	X
Neonates	X	X											
Age >75	X	X					X				X		
Cardiovascular disease							X	X		X	X		
Pulmonary disease										X	X		
Malignancy	X	X	(c)	(c)					X	X	X		
Radiation therapy		X							X				
Hepatic disease				X					X				
Expose to hepatitis													
Renal disease	X	X		X		X	X						
Bleeding disorder				X	X								X
Diabetes						X	X	X			X		
Smoking >20 pack/yr	X	X								X			
Diuretic use						X	X						
Digoxin						X	X				X		
Steriod use						X		X					
Anticoagulant use	X	X		X									
Central nervous system disease	X	X			X	X	X			X			
Possible pregnancy (d)													

Notes: (a) This is a simplified strategy which is not comprehensive. Therefore the clinician must use judgement regarding patients and conditions which are not listed.
(b) For minimally invasive surgery no tests other than those indicated for other medical care of the patient are needed.
(c) Obtain for leukaemias.
(d) Pregnancy test.
X, obtain test; Hb, haemoglobin; WBC, white blood cell count; PT, prothrombin time; PTT, partial thromboplastin time; PLT, platelet count; BT, bleeding time; ELECT, serum electrolytes; Cr, creatinine; BUN, blood urea nitrogen; SGOT, serum glutamic-oxaloacetic transaminase; ALK P, alkaline phosphatase; CXR, chest radiograph; ECG, electrocardiogram; ALB, albumin; T/S, blood type and antibody screen

minimising usage (whether based on avoidance of unneeded tests or for economic incentives) to one of optimising resource utilisation. We are responsible for ensuring that our patients get the best preparation possible and must act as their advocates.

The preoperative clinic itself is often seen only as a cost centre with minimal direct revenue generated when reviewed by hospital accountants. They must include an analysis of changes in other resources, such as tests, consultations, and operating room efficiency.

Summary

Table 3.3 presents a simplified strategy for preoperative testing.[38] This strategy is not static; rather, it is dynamic. There are many areas where the recommendations are based on limited data and expert judgement and there are many opportunities for improvement. Additionally, the triage of patients for preoperative evaluation and testing will be an active area of research as we move forward.

What has been clearly demonstrated is the benefit afforded by the considered interaction of an anaesthesiologist in obtaining a history and exam, with an eye to the planned procedure, and the subsequent application of the information gathered therein to plan a successful anaesthetic programme for each patient.

1   Gibby G, Gravenstein J, Layon A et al. How often does the preoperative interview change anaesthetic management? Anesthesiology 1992; 77: A1134.
2   Fischer SP. Development and effectiveness of an anesthesia preoperative evaluation clinic in a teaching hospital [see comments]. Anesthesiology 1996; 85: 196–206.
3   Vacanti CJ, van Houten RJ, Hill RC. A statistical analysis of the relationship of physical status to postoperative mortality in 68,388 cases. Anesth Analg 1970; 49: 564–6.
4   Lewin I, Lerner AG, Green SH, Del GL, Siegel J. Physical class and physiologic status in the prediction of operative mortality in the aged sick. Ann Surg 1971; 174: 217–31.
5   Goldman L, Caldera DL, Nussbaum SR et al. Multifactorial index of cardiac risk in noncardiac surgical procedures. N Engl J Med 1977; 297: 845–50.
6   Chung F, Mezei G, Tong D. Pre-existing medical conditions as predictors of adverse events in day-case surgery. Br J Anaesth 1999; 83: 262–70.
7   Fowkes FG, Lunn JN, Farrow SC, Robertson IB, Samuel P. Epidemiology in anaesthesia. III: Mortality risk in patients with coexisting physical disease. Br J Anaesth 1982; 54: 819–25.
8   Pasternak L. Preanesthesia evaluation of the surgical patient. In: ASA annual refresher course lectures. Hagersdown: American Society of Anesthesiologists, 1996: 205.
9   Schein OD, Katz J, Bass EB et al. The value of routine preoperative medical testing before cataract surgery. N Engl J Med 2000; 342: 168–75.
10 Haug RH, Reifeis RL. A prospective evaluation of the value of preoperative laboratory testing for office anesthesia and sedation. J Oral Maxillofac Surg 1999; 57: 16–20; discussion 21–2.
11 Manley S, de Kelaita G, Joseph NJ, Salem MR, Heyman HJ. Preoperative pregnancy testing in ambulatory surgery. Incidence and impact of positive results [see comments]. Anesthesiology 1995; 83: 690–3.
12 Burke DS, Brundage JF, Redfield RR et al. Measurement of the false positive rate in a screening program for human immunodeficiency virus infections. N Engl J Med 1988; 319: 961–4.

13   Mangano DT. Perioperative cardiac morbidity. *Anesthesiology* 1990; **72**: 153–84.

14   Eagle KA, Brundage BH, Chaitman BR *et al.* Guidelines for perioperative cardiovascular evaluation for noncardiac surgery. Report of the American College of Cardiology/ American Heart Association Task Force on Practice Guidelines. Committee on Perioperative Cardiovascular Evaluation for Noncardiac Surgery [see comments]. *Circulation* 1996; **93**: 1278–317.

15   Koenig W, Sund M, Frohlich M *et al.* C-reactive protein, a sensitive marker of inflammation, predicts future risk of coronary heart disease in initially healthy middle-aged men: results from the MONICA (Monitoring Trends and Determinants in Cardiovascular Disease) Augsburg Cohort Study, 1984 to 1992. *Circulation* 1999; **99**: 237–42.

16   Ridker PM, Buring JE, Shih J, Matias M, Hennekens CH. Prospective study of C-reactive protein and the risk of future cardiovascular events among apparently healthy women [see comments]. *Circulation* 1998; **98**: 731–3.

17   Rohde LE, Hennekens CH, Ridker PM. Survey of C-reactive protein and cardiovascular risk factors in apparently healthy men. *Am J Cardiol* 1999; **84**: 1018–22.

18   McKee RF, Scott EM. The value of routine preoperative investigations. *Ann R Coll Surg Engl* 1987; **69**: 160.

19   Rabkin SW, Horne JM. Preoperative electrocardiography: its cost-effectiveness in detecting abnormalities when a previous tracing exists. *Can Med Assoc J* 1979; **121**: 301.

20   Rabkin SW, Horne JM. Preoperative electrocardiography: effect of new abnormalities on clinical decisions. *Can Med Assoc J* 1983; **128**: 146.

21   Detsky AS, Abrams HB, McLaughlin JR *et al.* Predicting cardiac complications in patients undergoing non-cardiac surgery. *J Gen Intern Med* 1986; **1**: 211–19.

22   Berthe C, Pierard LA, Hiernaux M *et al.* Predicting the extent and location of coronary artery disease in acute myocardial infarction by echocardiography during dobutamine infusion. *Am J Cardiol* 1986; **58**: 1167–72.

23   Cohen JL, Greene TO, Ottenweller J, Binenbaum SZ, Wilchfort SD, Kim CS. Dobutamine digital echocardiography for detecting coronary artery disease. *Am J Cardiol* 1991; **67**: 1311–18.

24   Tape TG, Mushlin AI. How useful are routine chest X-rays of preoperative patients at risk for postoperative chest disease? *J Gen Intern Med* 1988; **3**: 15–20.

25   Wasserman LR, Gilbert HS. Surgical bleeding in polycythemia vera. *Ann NY Acad Sci* 1964; **115**: 122.

26   Weiskopf RB, Viele MK, Feiner J *et al.* Human cardiovascular and metabolic response to acute, severe isovolemic anemia. *JAMA* 1998; **279**: 217.

27   Carson JL, Duff A, Berlin JA. Perioperative blood transfusion and postoperative mortality. *JAMA* 1998; **279**: 199.

28   de Caterina R, Lanza M, Manca G, Strata GB, Maffei S, Salvatore L. Bleeding time and bleeding: an analysis of the relationship of the bleeding time test with parameters of surgical bleeding. *Blood* 1994; **84**: 3363–70.

29   Suchman AL, Mushlin AI. How well does the activated partial thromboplastin time predict postoperative hemorrhage? *JAMA* 1986; **256**: 750–3.

30   Macpherson DS. Preoperative laboratory testing: should any tests be "routine" before surgery? *Med Clin North Am* 1993; 77: 289.

31   Steiner A, Weisser B, Vetter W. A comparative review of the adverse effects of treatments for hyperlipidaemia. *Drug Saf* 1991; **6**: 118–30.

32   Hirsh IA, Tomlinson DL, Slogoff S *et al.* The overstated risk of preoperative hypokalemia. *Anesth Analg* 1988; **67**: 131.

33   Vitez TS, Soper LE, Wong KC *et al.* Chronic hypokalemia and intraoperative dysrhythmias. *Anesthesiology* 1985; **63**: 130.

34   Cooper JW. Adverse drug reactions and interactions in a nursing home. *Nurs Homes Sr Citiz Care* 1987; **36**: 7–11.

35   Lawson DH. Adverse reactions to potassium chloride. *Quart J Med* 1974; **43**: 433.

36   Macario A, Roizen MF, Thisted RA, Kim S, Orkin FK, Phelps C. Reassessment of preoperative laboratory testing has changed the test-ordering patterns of physicians. *Surg Gynecol Obstet* 1992; **175**: 539–47.

37   Roizen MF, Kaplan EB, Schreider BD, Lichtor LJ, Orkin FK. The relative roles of the history and physical examination, and laboratory testing in preoperative evaluation for outpatient surgery: the "Starling" curve of preoperative laboratory testing. *Anesthesiol Clin North Am* 1987; 5: 15–34.
38   Roizen M, Foss J, Fischer S. Preoperative evaluation. In: Miller R, ed. *Anesthesia,* Vol 1, 5th edn. Philadelphia: Churchill Livingstone, 1999: 824–83.

4: Implications of intercurrent disease

LESLEY M BROMLEY

Introduction

In the first Confidential Enquiry into Perioperative Deaths (CEPOD)[1] report published in 1989, the section on anaesthesia described a subset of patients where death was anaesthesia related. These deaths constituted 14.1% of the deaths in the study, but in only three deaths was anaesthesia recorded as the sole factor responsible for death; two of these deaths related to inability to secure the airway. In the remaining 407 deaths where anaesthesia played a part, the assessors were not satisfied with the preoperative preparation of patients in 25% of cases.

The incidence of intercurrent disease in the anaesthesia related deaths group was similar to that in the whole CEPOD sample. The commonest disease states were those affecting the cardiovascular and respiratory systems, with diabetes mellitus and rheumatoid arthritis also figuring significantly. There were 850 different disease processes recorded in 410 patients, reflecting the fact that patients often had more than one intercurrent disease. The CEPOD assessors considered 18% of the deaths in this category to have been avoidable. In one-third of cases it was deemed that the assessment and preparation of the patient before operation had been inadequate and that the implications of intercurrent disease had not been appreciated. Intercurrent disease was highlighted as a contributory factor to death in 51% of anaesthetic-related deaths and as the sole factor in 22% of deaths.

Clearly the risk associated with anaesthesia is increased by intercurrent disease, but the emphasis of the CEPOD report is that the patient with intercurrent disease that is not optimally treated at the time of surgery is subject to even greater risk. It is noteworthy that much of the risk assessment literature is based on the risk to a patient who has his or her disease optimally treated.

In broad terms the classification of physical status defined by the American Society of Anesthesiologists (ASA), used commonly throughout anaesthesia and surgery, has been shown to be a good predictor of postoperative outcome (Box 4.1).

Box 4.1 American Society of Anesthesiologists classification of Physical Status

ASA 1	Normal healthy patient
ASA II	Patient with mild-to-moderate systemic disease with no functional limitation
ASA III	Patient with severe systemic disease with definite limitation of normal function
ASA IV	Patient with severe systemic disease that is a constant threat to life
ASA V	Moribund patient unlikely to survive 24 h with or without operation

Addition of the letter "E" indicates that surgery is to be undertaken as an emergency procedure

An increase in ASA category was associated with a stepwise 2–3-fold increase in postoperative complications. This included surgical complications such as wound infection as well as symptoms associated with intercurrent disease. An increase in ASA category also carried a stepwise 5–7-fold increase in in-hospital mortality.[2]

Implications of cardiovascular disease

Congestive cardiac failure, ischaemic heart disease, hypertension, atrial fibrillation, myocardial infarction, and cerebrovascular accident form the majority of the intercurrent diseases recorded by CEPOD. These diseases are indeed very common in the general population and the key question relating to them is the extent to which anaesthesia will exacerbate the disease process. Cardiovascular complication rates of 2–6% occur in many reports of postoperative complications, although death from cardiovascular causes is less common; one study of 17 201 patients undergoing general anaesthesia recorded 19 deaths and 23 myocardial infarctions.[3] In general, deaths from cardiac causes are defined as death from myocardial infarction, from cardiac failure or from cerebrovascular accident. These low numbers require the study of large populations to identify the risk factors and understand their implications.

The risk factors for cardiovascular events in the postoperative period have been identified. In particular, five preexisting conditions have been found to be significant risk factors for cardiac death in patients undergoing elective surgery: a history of myocardial infarction, angina, hypertension, heart failure, and renal failure. Further analysis indicates that myocardial infarction and renal failure are the most significant of these. Angina in the absence of a previous myocardial infarction is also significant.[4]

The importance of a history of hypertension as a risk factor for elective surgery is less clear. In some studies poorly controlled hypertension was

59

associated with intraoperative cardiovascular instability and ischaemia. Thus Browner and colleagues[5] found an association between a history of hypertension and mortality after major non-cardiac surgery whereas several studies, including that of Goldman and colleagues,[6] have found no such association. It appears that statistical analysis of risk factors by univariate or multivariate analysis in a variety of populations produces an association between hypertension and adverse cardiac outcome which is on the borders of significance, appearing in some studies but not in others. In contrast, previous myocardial infarction and renal failure are consistently identified in all studies. Heart failure becomes more significant if there is no previous myocardial infarction. This underlines the fact that the state of the myocardium is the risk factor and that the manifestation of its dysfunction varies.

The risk of mortality is greater with urgent or emergency surgery, whilst co-morbidity may be more significant when combined with the surgical condition. Fowkes and colleagues reported a mortality of 1.5 per 100 elective cases, but 5.3 per 100 emergency cases.[7] Comparable incidences of postoperative complications occur in elective and emergency cases but the incidence of adverse outcomes is greater in emergency cases. In the patient about to undergo an emergency procedure the most significant cardiovascular risk arises from co-existing heart failure. The presence of heart failure and previous myocardial infarction within the previous year are major determinants of intra- and postoperative complications, whilst chronic heart failure is of major importance for in-hospital death. Renal failure is also a risk factor for perioperative cardiovascular death in emergency patients. This may represent, in addition to underlying pathology, inadequate resuscitation of the emergency patient.

Hypertension was not identified as a risk factor for morbidity or mortality in emergency surgery. The interpretation of this factor must be influenced by the fact that many patients about to undergo emergency surgery will be hypotensive as a result of fluid depletion from third-space losses or vomiting or because of underresuscitation. Where patients who were hypertensive at the time of emergency surgery were examined in detail, cardiovascular complications occurred in 42% and the mortality was 22%.[8]

Preexisting cardiovascular disease increases the morbidity and mortality from anaesthesia and surgery. The incidence of cardiac death following anaesthesia is low, but where it occurs, it is statistically likely to be associated with previous myocardial infarction, renal failure and, in the emergency case, cardiac failure. Other manifestations of ischaemic heart disease and hypertension are all indications that the cardiovascular system is at risk but they are not statistically significant risk factors. Hypertension is a borderline risk factor, positive in some studies but not in others. In emergency surgery the presence of hypertension appears to be associated with a high incidence of morbidity and mortality.

Implications of respiratory disease

Respiratory disease is common in the UK population and patients often suffer from both cardiac and respiratory disease.[9] Cigarette smoking is a common factor in a large number of patients. Inhalational anaesthetic agents have a number of profound effects on respiratory function in the peri- and postoperative period. It is therefore no surprise that respiratory disease influences outcome from general anaesthesia. The use of regional anaesthesia, if appropriate, may reduce the impact of anaesthesia and surgery on the patient with respiratory disease.[10]

Chronic obstructive pulmonary disease (COPD) varies in its severity from chronic production of sputum through to significantly reduced forced expiratory volume in one second (FEV_1) and FEV_1/ FVC (forced vital capacity) ratio. It has been shown that patients with a FEV_1 of equal to or less than 1.2 litres are at greater risk of postoperative pulmonary complications.[11] This would be in the region of 50% less than the predicted value for FEV_1. The common complications experienced by these patients are atelectasis and pneumonia, resulting in prolonged mechanical ventilation and prolonged intensive care stay.[12] Respiratory failure and death are less common; in a large sample of all patients undergoing routine surgery, respiratory failure occurred eight times in 13 693 anaesthetics.[3]

Patients who have severe COPD are at greater risk of all these complications. Shapiro and colleagues have devised a classification of risk of pulmonary complications for abdominal and thoracic procedures, which includes respiratory spirography, arterial blood gases and factors relating to cardiac and nervous system function (Table 4.1).[13]

An elevated Shapiro score and ASA category and the need to perform abdominal surgery, particularly emergency abdominal surgery, were associated with both a high mortality and a high incidence of pulmonary complications. Patients with severe COPD have a poor long-term survival after anaesthesia; a two-year follow-up of such patients reported a mortality rate of 47%.[14] In the same study the perioperative deaths were confined to patients who had an FEV_1 of less than 750 ml and a Shapiro score of greater than 5. However, consideration of the type and duration of surgery in patients with COPD is important in looking at the overall outcome for these patients.

Although there are a relatively small number of patients with such severe respiratory disease, there are a very large number of patients who smoke tobacco, usually cigarettes, in some form or another. The risks of smoking in relation to the development of heart disease, cancers, and chronic lung disease are well known but the smoker is also at higher risk from anaesthesia. Perioperative respiratory complications such as intubation problems, need for reintubation, laryngospasm, bronchospasm, aspiration, hypoventilation, and hypoxaemia are all more common in smokers than

Table 4.1 Classification of risk of pulmonary complications of thoracic and abdominal procedures (reproduced with permission from reference[13])

	Category	Points
I	*Respiratory system*	
A.	Normal expiratory spirogram ie %FVC + %FEV$_1$/FVC > 150	0
B.	%FVC + %FEV$_1$/FVC = 100–150	1
C.	%FVC + %FEV$_1$/FVC 100	2
D.	Preoperative FVC < 20mL/kg	3
E.	Post-bronchodilator FEV$_1$/FVC<50%	3
II	*Cardiovascular system*	
A.	Normal	0
B.	Controlled hypertension, myocardial infarction, without sequelae for more than 2 years	0
C.	Dyspnoea on exertion, orthopnoea, paroxysmal nocturnal dyspnoea, dependent oedema, congestive heart failure, angina	1
III	*Nervous system*	
A.	Normal	0
B.	Confusion, obtunded, agitation, spasticity, discoordination, bulbar malfunction	1
C.	Significant muscular weakness	1
IV	*Arterial blood gases*	
A.	Acceptable	0
B.	Paco$_2$>50 mm Hg or Pao$_2$<60 mm Hg on room air	1
C.	Metabolic pH abnormality > 7.5 or <7.3	1
V	*Postoperative ambulation*	
A.	Expected ambulation (minimum sitting at bedside) within 36 hours	0
B.	Expected complete confinement to bed for at least 36 hours	1

FEV^1, forced expiratory volume in one second; FVC, forced vital capacity
A maximum total score of 7 is possible

non-smokers.[15] The vast majority of these events cause no long-term morbidity that can be recognised but they are all potentially life threatening. The combination of chronic lung disease and smoking in young age groups carries a very high relative risk of perioperative bronchospasm. This perhaps reflects the fact that chronic lung disease is very rare and likely to be severe when it occurs in young people.

Asthma is the most common respiratory disease in the younger age groups and is increasing in incidence every year. Currently 4–5% of the population are asthmatic and asthma is now the leading chronic disease of childhood.[16] The prevalence and mortality of asthma have risen worldwide in the last decade. The manifestations of acute asthma, a variable airway obstruction accompanied by wheezing, can be precipitated by various aspects of anaesthesia. Thus manipulating the airway can cause bronchospasm in the non-asthmatic patient. However, the asthmatic patient has hyperreactive bronchiolar smooth muscle and will be more sensitive to the effects of such manoeuvres. The treated asthmatic remains more sensitive than the normal individual but is less likely to suffer from perioperative exacerbations than the poorly treated individual.[17] Many of the drugs used in anaesthesia release histamine and this may further complicate the management of asthmatic patients.[18] When asthmatic patients are assessed for anaesthesia, they may be physically quite well with no wheeze on examination. In this event the history of previous attacks and their management and the bronchodilator therapy used are important indicators of the severity of the disease. Intraoperative acute bronchospam may result in profound hypoxia. However, the anaesthetised patient is able to receive prompt treatment as the airway is secure and the patient unconscious. If treatment is rapid no long-term sequelae will result.

A common precipitant of wheezing in the asthmatic patient is the presence of an upper respiratory tract infection (URTI). In the non-asthmatic patient severe URTI may produce some chest signs such as rhonchi and rales. In the winter months many patients will present with developing or resolving URTIs. The significance of these infections in terms of outcome from anaesthesia is important. URTIs affect the airway from the nose down to the small airways and the lung parenchyma. During the period of toxic viraemia the patient is pyrexial. The presence of pyrexia with URTI symptoms is a contraindication for elective anaesthesia.[19] Risks associated with anaesthesia in this period include perioperative airways obstruction, laryngospasm, and vagally mediated reflex bronchoconstriction with arterial desaturation. In the postoperative period atelectasis and chest infections are more common.[20]

In addition to these respiratory complications, the occasional death associated with an undiagnosed viral myocarditis accompanying an URTI does occur. This seems to be more common in young adults. The incidence of perioperative respiratory complications remains higher for six weeks after the resolution of the pyrexia.[21] This poses a particular problem in paediatric anaesthesia. Children suffer from runny noses, colds, and coughs more frequently than do adults. When a child presents for a procedure under anaesthesia the implications of cancellation are widespread for both the family and the institution. Who then should be cancelled? Clearly any child with a temperature, but many children will have runny noses all the time. The consensus opinion of the published literature is that children with moderate-to-severe symptoms of a respiratory tract infection should have their operation cancelled for six weeks, but if symptoms are mild and have not worsened in the previous few days, anaesthesia can proceed with caution. Nevertheless, emergency surgery may have to be performed in patients with URTIs, in which case careful postoperative monitoring is required.

There are many other conditions of the airway, lung, and chest wall which are less common than COPD and asthma. Any lung disease can complicate anaesthesia. Restrictive disease may present problems for mechanical ventilation. Bullous disease will increase the risk of pneumothorax when intermittent positive pressure ventilation is used. Diseases of the chest wall and the musculature may complicate the return to spontaneous breathing after anaesthesia and require prolonged ventilation.

Obstructive sleep apnoea, a condition that occurs in 2% of the population, has implications for anaesthesia and is commonly undiagnosed.[22] Patients have frequent periods of apnoea and arterial desaturation during normal sleep. In the postoperative period these events may be worsened by the use of opiate analgesics and arterial desaturations as low as 50% accompanied by cardiac arrhythmias can occur. A number of deaths have been reported.[23]

Implications of endocrine disease

The commonly occurring endocrine diseases that are important for anaesthesia are diabetes mellitus and thyrotoxicosis. Progress in the management of these two conditions has reduced their importance as causes of anaesthetic morbidity. The long-term consequences of these diseases remain significant to anaesthesia.

Diabetes mellitus

Diabetes mellitus is a systemic disease with many long-term complications. Its immediate management in the postoperative period is now well described and the advent of accurate bedside blood glucose estimation has greatly aided accurate maintenance of the blood sugar in the operative period.[24] During anaesthesia, hypoglycaemia is potentially more dangerous than hyperglycaemia as its symptoms may be misinterpreted as lightening of the level of anaesthesia. The use of diagnostic "sticks" and glucometers for blood sugar estimation has enabled rapid differentiation and greatly enhanced safety for diabetic patients. A history of poor control with frequent episodes of hypoglycaemia is therefore of significance and indicates the need for extra vigilance.

The long-term sequelae of diabetes mellitus are themselves important for anaesthesia. The high incidence of ischaemic heart disease, hypertension, and renal failure in long-term diabetic patients increases their risks of peri- and postoperative complications. Mortality and morbidity from surgery are higher in diabetics than in non-diabetics.[25] In the many analyses of operative and anaesthetic risk that have been performed, diabetes itself is not a predictive risk factor but the complications of long-term diabetes occur frequently in these predictive models. Thus good diabetic control in the past and over the operative period will result in little or no extra risk to the patient.

The stress of surgery makes diabetic control more difficult and higher blood sugars may promote wound infections.[26] Neuropathic conditions may develop; sensory neuropathy makes the patient vulnerable to damage to the limbs during positioning whereas autonomic neuropathy may cause cardiovascular complications during intermittent positive pressure ventilation.[27]

Some diabetic patients suffer from the "stiff joint syndrome" in which joint contractures and a thickening of the skin are associated with rapidly progressing microvascular disease. These patients may be difficult to intubate. Diabetic patients undergoing anaesthesia have a higher incidence of difficult laryngoscopy, associated with strictures in the anterior part of the larynx. This syndrome has been identified in diabetic patients undergoing renal transplantation, reflecting the complications of poor diabetic control.[28]

Thyroid disease

Thyrotoxicosis should be controlled before anaesthesia is undertaken. The risk of precipitating a thyroid crisis is greater in the poorly controlled patient. Thyroid crisis, although uncommon, can result in tachyarrhythmias and cardiac failure.[29] Thyrotoxicosis can be difficult to diagnose in the pregnant patient and the symptoms may be masked by β-blockade where the first presentation may be circulatory collapse. These events are rare, but have significant morbidity when they occur.[30]

Implications of gastrointestinal and liver disease

Alimentary tract

Disorders of the upper gastrointestinal (GI) tract that make aspiration of gastric contents into the lung more likely are of significance. The presence of symptoms of acid regurgitation and "heartburn" particularly on lying down or leaning forwards, would be important considerations for anaesthesia. The underlying disease process for these symptoms may be multifactorial. Pregnancy, obesity, achalasia of the oesophagus, strictures, and tumours of the oesophagus may all produce these symptoms. Appropriate measures are required to reduce the risk of pulmonary aspiration of gastric contents.[31] Delay in gastric emptying can be produced by a number of circumstances, such as drugs (for example, opiates), pain, the content of the meal, and obstruction of the small intestine. These may all contribute to a full stomach after the expected period for emptying. The full stomach is also more likely to result in regurgitation at induction of anaesthesia regardless of the state of the oesophagus. Conditions that increase gastric acid secretion will also increase the risk of anaesthesia. These are fortunately rare and are now well controlled by drug therapy when diagnosed. See also Chapter 8.

Carcinoid syndrome is a rare syndrome associated with tumours of the gut. They arise most commonly from the mid-gut, one-third of them presenting in the appendix. About 25% of the tumours produce the syndrome, dependent on the secretion of 5-hydroxytryptamine and other tachykinins. The majority of patients with carcinoid will have hepatic metastases. Treatment with somatostatin analogues has greatly improved the outcome from surgery but the tumours often recur.[32]

Disorders of the lower GI tract are rarely significant for anaesthesia, but obstruction of the small or large bowel, subacute or acute, has great significance. Disorders of fluid and electrolyte balance which result must be corrected before surgery. Bowel obstruction requiring surgery is one of the commonest surgical emergencies. The optimisation of the cardiovascular system in such patients before surgery is undertaken has a profound effect on the outcome from surgery. Bowel resection may be required as a matter of urgency but time spent on correcting fluids and electrolytes may be life saving and should be performed before as well as during anaesthesia.[33]

Liver disease

The most significant diseases of the GI tract are those of the liver. Symptomatic liver disease has several implications for anaesthesia and surgery. The reduction in synthetic functions of the liver results in reduced clotting factors and reduced plasma proteins for binding with drugs. The ability of the liver to metabolise anaesthetic drugs may be impaired. The presence of obstructive jaundice may be associated with the hepatorenal syndrome in which renal failure complicates the hepatic failure.[34] Bleeding from oesophageal varices indicates significant hepatic disease. The common aetiologies of hepatic failure are chronic hepatitis and alcohol abuse. Chronic hepatitis carried a risk of infecting theatre staff that must be considered. The vast majority of theatre staff are vaccinated against hepatitis B but as yet there is no anti-hepatitis C vaccine. Chronic alcohol abuse may be accompanied by alcoholic cardiomyopathy.

Hepatic resection may be undertaken for the removal of hepatic metastases from primary carcinomas elsewhere; these operations may require extensive blood and clotting factor transfusion.

Implications of renal disease

Chronic renal failure is a progression from reduced glomerular filtration rate, decreased renal reserve, renal insufficiency through to end-stage renal failure. All but the last of these conditions can be made worse by anaesthesia and surgery. Potential reduction in renal blood flow and drug-induced nephrotoxicity can accompany anaesthesia.[35] Ideally the patient should be dialysed immediately prior to anaesthesia. However, this may not be possible. If the surgery is to establish a route for dialysis the renal status of the patient may be severely deranged. Patients in chronic renal failure presenting for emergency treatment may have to undergo surgery before dialysis can be performed. By contrast, renal transplantation is carried out on patients who have been dialysed electively.

Patients in renal failure are commonly hypertensive and have a hyperdynamic circulation. This latter effect is a combination of chronic anaemia and uraemic cardiomyopathy. The anaemia of chronic renal failure is minimised by the use of erythropoietin, but this does not completely correct the abnormality and these patients have a low haemoglobin level.[36] These effects lead to left ventricular failure. In addition, there is an increased incidence of coronary artery disease and cerebrovascular accidents in patients with end-stage renal failure. If dialysis has not been performed recently there is a significant risk of fluid overload and pulmonary oedema. There is also an increased susceptibility to chest infections. Thus chronic renal failure results in an increased incidence of cardiac risk factors for anaesthesia.

The presence of a high serum urea has a number of effects on the patient, including a delay in gastric emptying and an increase in acid secretion in the stomach.[37] These increase the risk of gastric aspiration at induction of anaesthesia. Uraemia alters the binding of many anaesthetic drugs, making their titration more difficult. Patients in chronic renal failure may have autonomic neuropathy; this may be reversed after renal transplantation[38]

Patients with end-stage renal failure who have been dialysed can be difficult to anaesthetise. The circulation is often brittle and vasodilator anaesthetic drugs may produce a profound reduction in blood pressure, while reducing the anaesthetic agent may then increase the risk of awareness. For this reason, where possible, regional techniques should be used.[39]

Renal failure increases the risk of anaesthesia directly and indirectly because of the complications of the disease. Patients who have undergone renal transplantation have many of the adverse effects reversed but if they have waited a long time for their transplant the cardiovascular changes will be irreversible. Renal failure, in a similar fashion to diabetes, is not a primary predictor of cardiovascular complications in multivariate analyses but is a secondary factor.[40]

Implications of rheumatoid arthritis

Rheumatoid arthritis is a systemic disease and has many manifestations that can complicate anaesthesia.[41] It primarily affects the joints with inflammatory damage leading to joint deformation and destruction. Half the affected patients also have extraarticular manifestations in the lungs, kidneys, and cardiovascular system.

Involvement of the cervical vertebrae is probably the most significant change of importance for anaesthesia. Instability of these joints, which may be asymptomatic, occurs in 25% of patients with rheumatoid arthritis. The danger of manipulating the neck under anaesthesia in such patients is of producing damage to the cervical cord. Atlantoaxial subluxation with compression of the cord by the odontoid peg against the arch of the atlas is the commonest lesion.[42] Many patients with symptomatic cervical vertebral disease undergo occipital cervical fusion. Unfortunately, they may develop further instabilities below the level of the arthrodesis. The fusion of the upper cervical vertebrae, whilst providing some neck stability, will itself contribute to difficulty in intubation of these subjects. Other joints in the head and neck may be affected, mouth opening may be limited and the joints of the larynx itself may be involved. All of these symptoms contribute to an increased risk of difficult intubation in the presence of a potentially unstable cervical column.[43]

The extraarticular manifestations of the disease are also of significance. Juvenile rheumatoid arthritis and ankylosing spondylitis are both associated with cardiac problems. Pericardial effusions, conduction abnormalities due to involvement of His–Purkinje fibres, and aortic valve involvement, sometimes of acute onset, have been recorded.[44] Cardiac tamponade from a rheumatoid pericardial effusion can occur.[45] The lungs may be affected by effusions, nodular lesions, and diffuse interstitial fibrosis, all reducing pulmonary reserve. Involvement of the intercostovertebral joints may produce a restrictive lung defect. Renal infiltration from the disease, from amyloidosis or from the nephrotoxic effects of the antirheumatoid drugs results in end-stage renal failure in 25% of patients with rheumatoid arthritis. Twenty of the anaesthesia-related deaths reported to CEPOD were in patients with rheumatoid arthritis.

Atlantoaxial instability is also a feature of Down's syndrome. This may be asymptomatic, but radiographic examination of children with Down's syndrome has shown that up to 20% have abnormalities of the cervical vertebrae.[46] Long-term outcome of arthrodesis of the cervical spine has been disappointing.[47] Down's syndrome is also associated with various cardiac abnormalities: septal defects, tetralogy of Fallot, and patent ductus arteriosus are all common.

Implications of pregnancy

Pregnancy is not a disease but an altered physiological state. Most women embarking on pregnancy are young and healthy. Pregnancy does have some implications for anaesthesia. The changes associated with pregnancy develop over the period of the pregnancy and persist for up to six weeks after delivery. Hormonal changes start from six weeks postconception. In the first trimester 30% of patients suffer from heartburn, indicating a higher risk of acid aspiration. As the pregnancy develops the effects of the developing uterus and fetus cause changes to respiratory function, raise intraabdominal pressure, and reduce the lower oesophageal barrier pressure.[48] Aortocaval compression by the uterus can be seen in the second trimester and becomes increasingly significant as term is approached.[49]

Cardiac output increases in the second and third trimester and the intravascular volume is increased. The pregnant woman has a high circulating plasma volume and has relatively low haemoglobin and plasma protein levels. At term the pregnant woman may be more difficult to intubate; about 1:300 obstetric general anaesthetics are said to be difficult intubations.[50] In part, this is because of mechanical difficulties; the procedure is often an emergency and cricoid pressure used to prevent aspiration may make intubation more difficult if it is overenthusiastically applied.

Some pregnant women present with co-existing disease; diabetes mellitus, cardiac disease, asthma, neurological and autoimmune diseases all co-exist with pregnancy. The management of these patients can present serious obstetric challenges. Congenital heart disease, heart/lung transplants, cardiomyopathies, and dysrhythmias all complicate about 1:350 pregnancies. Patients with Eisenmenger's syndrome have a 50% mortality in pregnancy. About 1:100 pregnant women are asthmatic, of whom 25% will deteriorate in pregnancy and will need aggressive treatment. Rheumatoid arthritis occurs in 1:1000 pregnancies and systemic lupus erythematosus (SLE) in 1:1600; the additional complication of rheumatoid changes in the neck with the difficult intubation caused by pregnancy means that operative delivery under general anaesthesia may entail a considerable risk for these patients.[51]

Twenty-five percent of pregnant women will develop some symptoms of preeclampsia during their pregnancy. Only 2% will have severe disease, the majority having symptoms of mild hypertension and peripheral oedema. The disease is more common in first pregnancies (75% of all preeclampsia) and in multiple pregnancy. Where it occurs in a second pregnancy, it is associated with the development of early cardiac disease in the mother. In severe preeclampsia the patient has a high systemic vascular resistance and a low colloid osmotic pressure. Infusion of relatively low volumes of fluid can produce pulmonary oedema. Oliguria may occur and renal function may be impaired for some months after delivery. The clotting may be disordered, there is a greater risk of complications from the pregnancy and of premature delivery of the baby.[52]

A variant on preeclampsia is the HELLP (haemolysis, elevated liver enzymes and low platelets) syndrome, in which hypertension may be mild but liver function is impaired and the platelet count is low. This syndrome is associated with pre-, inter- and postpartum haemorrhage.[53]

Implications of neurological disease

The central nervous system is an organ with integrating and coordinating functions which processes and responds to information received from the peripheral nervous system. Neurological disease may thus affect the peripheral nervous system and/or the central nervous system.

Diseases affecting the peripheral nervous system

Peripheral neuropathies are disorders of the structure and function of peripheral nerves. They may be acute (for example, Guillain–Barré syndrome), subacute or chronic and result in alterations in muscle tone, commonly hypotonicity. Hypertonicity, as with Parkinson's disease (see below), is also possible. Rapidly progressive peripheral neurological disease resulting in weakness of the bulbar muscles and muscles of respiration will necessitate urgent tracheal intubation and artificial ventilation if the vital capacity decreases to less than 15 ml/kg. A number of nutritional conditions (for example, vitamin B_{12} deficiency, alcohol-induced thiamine deficiency), metabolic conditions (for example, diabetes mellitus, uraemia, myxoedema) and toxic conditions (for example, heavy metals, some drugs) are associated with subacute and chronic neuropathies. Nerve degeneration is associated with changes in K^+ ion concentration and greatly exaggerated K^+ flux upon administration of suxamethonium.

Myasthenia gravis, a disease of myoneural transmission, is associated with excessive sensitivity to the effects of neuromuscular-blocking agents. Such drugs should be avoided if at all possible or used in very much reduced doses. Myasthenic patients will often be treated with immunosuppressive agents, including corticosteroids, and hence there is potential for drug–drug interactions. Muscular dystrophy and myotonia are diseases affecting the muscle fibres associated with continuing muscular contraction after voluntary effort has ceased. They are often associated with abnormalities of cardiac muscle, resulting in cardiac failure.

Diseases affecting the central nervous system

The significance of many diseases of the central nervous system (CNS) lies in the drugs used in their treatment. Migraine is one of the commonest conditions, affecting about 18% of women and 6% of men, with highest prevalence between the ages of 25 and 55 years.[54] However, drug therapy is rarely a problem for anaesthesia. This contrasts with epilepsy, another condition of the central nervous system that affects a proportion of the adult population. Pharmacotherapy for epilepsy may influence the metabolism of anaesthetic agents as a result of induction of hepatic enzymes or in their turn be affected by anaesthetic agents.

Parkinson's disease affects 1:100 people above the age of 55 years.[55] The mainstay of treatment are drugs which increase the synthesis and release of dopamine but which have potential for interaction with many of the drugs used in anaesthesia.

Multiple sclerosis (MS) is a complex trait characterised by relapses and remissions in which susceptibility is determined by both genetic and environmental factors.[56] General anaesthetics tend to be avoided in such patients due to concerns that they may exacerbate the condition. There is also a recognised association between MS and depression,[57] with potential for important interactions between antidepressant medication and anaesthetic agents (see below).

Acquired diseases of the CNS include infections (meningitis, encephalitis, and brain abscesses) and cerebral arterial disease. Cerebrovascular disease falls into two categories: occlusive and haemorrhagic. Occlusive cerebrovascular disease tends to occur in an older age group and is associated frequently with cardiovascular and other multisystem diseases. Haemorrhagic disease often has a congenital basis and occurs in younger age group.

Implications of psychiatric disease and psychological considerations in anaesthesia

Depression affects 5–6% of the population at any given time whilst 10% of the population will suffer from depression at some time during their lives. Therefore, it is likely that anaesthetists will encounter patients undergoing treatment for this condition. Although anaesthesia has no effect of itself on the course of a depressive illness, there may be potential drug interactions between antidepressant medication and anaesthetic agents. The same can also be said for schizophrenia, which affects 12% of the population. Patients with severe depression may present for anaesthesia for electroconvulsive treatment (ECT), in which case they should be assessed preoperatively for all intercurrent diseases in the same manner as for any other patient.[58]

Many patients have a fear of anaesthesia. This may be grounded in previous unpleasant experiences, for example a gaseous induction as a child or poorly managed postoperative pain. A small number of patients will have been aware during a previous general anaesthetic. The exact incidence of awareness is not known, as many patients do not report the experience to their doctor, but estimates based on structured interviews with postoperative patients suggest that between 1.2% and 0.2% of patients are aware during general anaesthesia.[59] In the past the incidence was probably higher as the introduction of anaesthetic agent monitoring in the operating theatre has allowed the anaesthetist to be reassured that the patient is receiving adequate anaesthesia. However, no good monitor of depth of anaesthesia is

71

available at the present time and as individual responses to the agents vary, there is still potential for awareness. Cardiac surgery and general anaesthetic caesarean sections were the operations during which awareness seems most likely to have occurred.

Patients who have had this experience may have long-lasting psychological problems. The most vulnerable to long-term sequelae are those who have been awake and not received adequate pain relief during surgery. These patients often have a morbid fear of hospitals, suffer from nightmares and flashbacks of the experience and may greatly benefit from psychological treatment.

Needle phobia, a morbid fear of hypodermic needle injections, is a growing problem. It occurs in patients who have had multiple treatments or operations, as well as in those who have never previously received an injection. It can arise as a result of unpleasant experiences in the dental surgery as well as in hospital. The need to gain venous access for safe induction of anaesthesia should be balanced against the psychological damage to the patient. The introduction of new anaesthetic vapours has allowed rapid gaseous induction as an alternative for these patients.

Anaesthesia for patients with special needs, particularly learning difficulties, represents a particular challenge. These patients are assessed from the point of view of their physical problems and in addition, they need careful psychological preparation by their carers and the medical team. They are best treated on a day case or short-stay basis, as the change of environment may be very upsetting to them. Carers are the best source of help and advice on the patient and the best way to achieve a smooth and atraumatic induction of anaesthesia.

Pharmacological considerations

Where patients are optimally treated for their intercurrent disease, consideration needs to be given to the drug treatment they are receiving. There is enormous potential for interaction between the drugs used to treat cardiac disease and the anaesthetic agents. In general, anaesthetic agents have a depressive effect on the cardiovascular system. The patient who is receiving cardiac and antihypertensive drugs should continue this treatment up to the morning of surgery, even into the period of fasting. The drugs should be taken with a small volume of water, at the normal time of day. The maintenance of these drugs is important as acute withdrawal combined with anaesthesia can produce unpredictable cardiovascular changes. The risks of such rebound phenomena far outweigh the risks of any interaction with anaesthetic agents.[60]

The calcium channel-blocking drugs nifedipine and verapamil have specific interactions with the volatile anaesthetic agents and are of particular significance. They can be summative in their effects, requiring vigilance. As all these drugs are cardiodepressive, they will also affect the pharmacokinetics of other drugs given.[61]

Drugs that modify electrolyte balance may have significance for anaesthesia. Diuretics, steroids, and insulin can all alter potassium homeostasis with the potential for arrhythmias during anaesthesia. Some anaesthetic drugs produce hyperkalaemia, particularly suxamethonium, and this can impair cardiac conduction.

A number of drugs can alter the duration of action of muscle-relaxant drugs. This is commonly brought about by altering the electrolyte balance in the neuromuscular junction. Thus an increase in magnesium decreases activity at the junction. Magnesium salts and lithium can bring about this effect. In contrast, calcium salts have the opposite effect and drugs which increase plasma calcium will antagonise competitive muscle relaxants and calcium channel-blocking drugs will potentiate muscle relaxants. Changes in acid–base balance will also modify neuromuscular transmission. Antibiotic drugs of the aminoglycoside group can cause neuromuscular blockade and potentiate the effect of muscle relaxants used in anaesthesia.[62]

Anaesthetic agents are global central depressants of neuronal function and are therefore likely to be potentiated by any other centrally acting depressant drugs. Thus opiate analgesics, benzodiazepines, hypnotics, and tranquillisers will all potentiate anaesthesia. This is highly significant in the recovery period, where sedation may be long lasting, rather than during the period of anaesthesia where the patient is intensively monitored and combinations of such drugs are often used as part of the anaesthetic technique.[63]

1   Buck N, Devlin HB, Lunn JN. *The Report of a Confidential Enquiry into Perioperative Deaths*. London: King's Fund, 1989.
2   Wolters J, Wolf T, Stutzer H, Schroder T. ASA classification and perioperative variables as predictors of postoperative outcome. *Br J Anaesth* 1996; 77: 217–22.
3   Forrest JB, Rehder K, Goldsmith CH *et al*. Multicenter study of general anaesthesia. III: Predictors of severe perioperative adverse outcomes. *Anesthesiology* 1992; 76: 3–15.
4   Howell SJ, Sear YM, Yeates D *et al*. Risk factors for cardiovascular death after elective surgery under general anaesthesia. *Br J Anaesth* 1998; 80: 14–19.
5   Browner WS, Li J, Mangano DT. In hospital mortality in male veterans following noncardiac surgery. *JAMA* 1992; 268: 228–32.
6   Goldman L, Caldera DL, Nussbaum SR *et al*. Multifactorial index of cardiac risk in noncardiac surgical procedures. *N Engl J Med* 1997; 97: 845–50.
7   Fowkes FGR, Lunn JN, Farrow SC *et al*. Epidemiology in anaesthesia III. Mortality risk in patients with co-existing disease. *Br J Anaesth* 1982; 54: 819–25.
8   Tiret L, Hatton F. Prediction of outcome of anaesthesia in patients over 40 years: a multifactorial risk index. *Stat Med* 1988; 7: 947–54.
9   Pedersen T, Eliasen K, Henriksen E. A prospective study of the mortality associated with anaesthesia and surgery: risk indicators of mortality in hospital. *Acta Anaesthesiol Scand* 1990; 34: 176–82.
10 Hendolin H, Lahtinen J, Lansimies E *et al*. The effects of thoracic epidural analgesia on respiratory function after cholecystectomy. *Acta Anaesthesiol Scand* 1987; 31: 645–51.
11 Garibaldi RA, Britt MR, Coleman ML *et al*. Risk factors for postoperative pneumonia. *Am J Med* 1981; 70: 677–80.

12 Tarhan S, Moffitt EA, Sessler AD *et al.* Risk of anesthesia and surgery in patients with chronic bronchitis and chronic obstructive pulmonary disease. *Surgery* 1973; **74**: 720–6.

13 Shapiro BA, Harrison RA, Kacmarek RM, Eds. *Clinical applications of respiratory care,* 3rd edn. Chicago: Yearbook Publishers, 1985.

14 Wong DH, Weber EC, Schell MJ, Wong AB, Anderson CT, Barker SJ. Factors associated with post operative pulmonary complications in patients with severe chronic obstructive pulmonary disease. *Anesth Analg* 1995; **80**: 276–84.

15 Schwilk B, Bothner U, Schraag S, Georgieff M. Perioperative respiratory events in smokers and nonsmokers undergoing general anaesthesia. *Acta Anaesthesiol Scand* 1997; **41**: 348–55.

16 Burney PG. Asthma mortality in England and Wales. Evidence for a further increase, 1974–1984. *Lancet* 1986; **2**: 323–6.

17 Hirshman CA, Bergman NA. Factors influencing intrapulmonary airway calibre during anaesthesia. *Br J Anaesth* 1990; **65**: 30–42.

18 Fletcher SW, Flacke W, Alper MH. The actions of general anesthetic agents on tracheal smooth muscle. *Anesthesiology* 1968; **29**: 517–22.

19 Prause G, Ratzenhofer-Komenda B, Smolle-Juettner F *et al.* Operations on patients deemed unfit for operation and anaesthesia: what are the consequences? *Acta Anaesthesiol Scand* 1998; **42**: 316–22.

20 Mlinaric J, Matulic Z, Mikecin M. Incidence of hypoxaemia events during anaesthesia in children with upper respiratory tract infection. *Medica Jadertina* 1998; **28**: 23–9.

21 van der Walt J. Anaesthesia in children with viral respiratory tract infections. *Paed Anaesth* 1997; **7**: 353–4

22 Gaultier C. Clinical and therapeutic aspects of obstructive sleep apnoea syndrome in infants and children. *Sleep* 1992; **15**: S36–8.

23 Richmond KH, Wetmore RF, Baranak CC *et al.* Postoperative complications following tonsillectomy and adenoidectomy: who is at risk? *Int J Pediat Otorhinolaryngol* 1987; **13**: 117–24.

24 Alberti KG, Thomas DJ. Management of diabetes during surgery. *Br J Anaesth* 1979; **51**: 693–710.

25 Hjortrup A, Rasmussen BF, Kehlet H. Morbidity in diabetic and non-diabetic patients after major vascular surgery. *BMJ* 1983; **287**: 1107–8.

26 McMurry FJ Jr. Wound healing with diabetes mellitus. Better glucose control for better wound healing in diabetics. *Surg Clin North Am* 1984; **64**: 769–78.

27 Page MM, Watkins PJ. Cardiorespiratory arrest and diabetic autonomic neuropathy. *Lancet* 1978; **i**: 14–16.

28 Salzarulo HH, Taylor LA. Diabetic 'stiff joint syndrome' as a cause of difficult endotracheal intubation. *Anesthesiology* 1986; **64**: 366–8.

29 Mackin JF, Canary JJ, Pittman CS. Thyroid storm and its management. *N Engl J Med* 1974; **291**: 1396–8.

30 Amino N, Morik H, Iwatani Y *et al.* High prevalence of transient post-partum thyrotoxicosis and hypothyroidism. *N Eng J Med* 1982; **306**: 849–52.

31 Warner MA, Warner ME, Webber JG. Clinical significance of pulmonary aspiration in the perioperative period. *Anesthesiology* 1993; **78**: 56–62.

32 Saini A, Waxman J. Management of carcinoid syndrome. *Postgrad Med J* 1991; **67**: 506–8.

33 Boyd O, Grounds RM, Bennett ED. A randomised clinical trial of the effect of deliberate perioperative increase of oxygen delivery on the mortality in high-risk surgical patients. *JAMA* 1983; **270**: 699–707.

34 Hishon S. The hepato-renal syndrome. *Hosp Update* 1981; **7**: 1027–35.

35 Maddern PJ. Anaesthesia for the patient with impaired renal function. *Anaesth Intens Care* 1983; **11**: 321–8.

36 MacDougall IC, Hutton RD, Cavill I *et al.* Treating renal anaemia with recombinant human erythropoietin: practical guidelines and a clinical algorithm. *BMJ* 1976; **300**: 655–8.

37 Weir PHC, Chung FF. Anaesthesia for chronic renal failure. *J Can Soc Anaesth* 1984; **31**: 468–80.

38 Graybar GB, Tarpley M. Kidney transplantation. In: Gelman S, ed. *Anesthesia and organ transplantation.* Philadelphia: WB Saunders 1987.

39   Eldredge SJ, Sperry R, Johnson JO. Regional anesthesia for arterio-venous fistula creation in the forearm: a new approach. *Anesthesiology* 1992; 77: 1230–1.

40   Aronson S, Blumenthal R. Perioperative renal dysfunction and cardiovascular anaesthesia: concerns and controversies. *J Cardiothorac Vasc Anaesth* 1998; 12: 567–86.

41   Khanam T. Anaesthetic risks in rheumatoid arthritis. *Br J Hosp Med* 1994; 52: 320–5.

42   Collins DN, Barnes CL, Fitzandolph RL. Cervical spine instability in rheumatoid patients having total hip or knee arthroplasty. *Clin Orthop* 1991; 272: 127–35.

43   Heywood AWB, Learmouth ID, Thomas M. Cervical spine instability in rheumatoid arthritis. *J Bone Joint Surg Br* 1988; 70: 702–7.

44   Camilleri JP, Douglas-Jones AG, Pitchard MH. Rapidly progressing aortic valve incompetence in a patient with rheumatoid arthritis. *Br J Rheumatol* 1991; 30: 379–81.

45   Burney DP, Martin CE, Thomas CS *et al.* Rheumatoid pericarditis. *J Thorac Cardiovasc Surg* 1979; 77: 511–15.

46   Konttinen YT, Santavirta S. Atlantoaxial instability in Down's syndrome *Lancet* 1989; i: 282.

47   Doyle JS, Lauerman WC, Wood KB, Krause DR. Complications and long-term outcome of upper cervical spine arthrodesis in patients with Down's syndrome. *Spine* 1996; 21: 1223–31.

48   Whitehead GM, Smith M, Dean Y, O'Sullivan G. An evaluation of gastric emptying times in pregnancy and the puerperium. *Anaesthesia* 1991; 48: 53–7.

49   James FM. Anaesthesia for non-obstetric surgery during pregnancy. *Clin Obstet Gynaecol* 1987; 30: 621–38.

50   Wilson ME, Speiglhalter D, Robertson JA, Lesser P. Predicting difficult intubation. *Br J Anaesth* 1988; 61: 211–16.

51   Ward ME, Douglas MJ. Medical aspects of obstetrics: diabetes, asthma, cardiac disease. *Curr Opin Anaesthesiol* 1993; 3: 483–6.

52   Robson SC, Redfern N, Walkinshaw S. A protocol for the interpartum management of severe pre-eclampsia. *Int J Obstet Anaesth* 1992; 1: 222–9.

53   Crosby TE. Obstetrical anaesthesia for patients with the syndrome of haemolysis, elevated liver enzymes, and low platelets. *Can J Anaesth* 1991; 38: 227–33.

54   Lipton RB, Stewart WF. Migraine headaches: epidemiology and comorbidity. *Clin Neurosci* 1998; 5: 2–9.

55   Hastings TG, Zigmond MJ. Loss of dopaminergic neurons in parkinsonism: possible role of reactive dopamine metabolites. *J Neural Transm* 1997; 49 *(suppl)*: 103–10.

56   Compston A. The genetic epidemiology of multiple sclerosis. *Philos Trans R Soc Lond B Biol Sci* 1999; 354: 1623–34.

57   Patten SB, Metz LM. Depression in multiple sclerosis. *Psychother Psychosom* 1997; 66: 286–92.

58   O'Flaherty D, Giesecke AH. Electroconvulsive therapy and anaesthesia. *Curr Opin Anaesthesiol* 1991; 4: 436–40.

59   Lui WHD, Thorp TAS, Graham SG, Aitkenhead AR. Incidence of awareness with recall during general anaesthesia. *Anaesthesia* 1991; 46: 435–7.

60   Goldman L, Caldera DL. Risk of general anesthesia and elective operation in the hypertensive patient. *Anesthesiology* 1979; 50: 285–92.

61   Merin RG, Chelly JE, Hysing ES *et al.* Cardiovascular effects of and interactions between calcium channel blocking drugs and anaesthetics in chronically instrumented dogs IV: chronically administered oral verapamil and halothane, enflurane, and isoflurane. *Anesthesiology* 1989; 66: 140–6.

62   Lee C, Katz RL. Neuromuscular pharmacology. *Br J Anaesth* 1980; 52: 173–88.

63   Perisho JA, Buechel DR, Millar RD *et al.* The effects of diazepam on minimum alveolar anaesthetic requirement in man. *Can Anaesth Soc J* 1979; 18: 536–40.

SECTION 2: Risk assessment

5: Assessing risk

JEAN-PIERRE VAN BESOUW

> "*Inquiry says surgeons should stop operating if patient dies.*"
>
> *BMJ*, 6th February 1999

In its broadest sense, "risk" is defined as the chance or probability of an adverse outcome.[1] In terms of the perioperative care of a patient, this can be further refined into risk of death or risk of an adverse outcome. The risk of death from any cause and for all cases in the perioperative period is around 1:1000. The incidence of anaesthetic-related causes of death is about 1:10 000 whilst the mortality rate for healthy patients undergoing day care surgery is around 1:22 000, both of which are less than that of driving a car.[2] Within the management of any one patient, the assessment of risk should be based on an analysis of both the patient and the health-care system responsible for the delivery of treatment, as the two are inextricably linked. It is beyond the scope of this chapter, however, to discuss these wider issues of assessing risk and it is my intention primarily to concentrate on the assessment of risk in the individual patient rather than on the institution or individuals delivering the care and the interactions between the two.

Quantifying risk

Risk assessment is the critical appraisal of what is potentially harmful, an assessment of its significance, and an evaluation of the measures available to eliminate or reduce that risk. The UK Health and Safety Executive (HSE), in their guide to employers on reducing risk in the workplace, suggest a five-step programme in order to minimise risk (Box 5.1).[3] The precepts outlined

Box 5.1 Assessment of risk in the workplace[3]

Step 1: Look for the hazards
Step 2: Decide who might be harmed
Step 3: Evaluate the risks and decide whether the existing precautions are adequate or whether more should be done
Step 4: Record findings
Step 5: Review assessment and revise where necessary

in this advice can be applied readily to the patient presenting for anaesthesia and surgery. Having identified at-risk individuals, risk control measures are aimed at reducing, preventing or avoiding any adverse events that could potentially occur. Anaesthetists should apply such an algorithm in their perioperative risk assessment of a patient.

Steps in the assessment of risk

Look for hazards

The process by which risk can be defined is dependent on a retrospective analysis of adverse outcomes for a given procedure. Adverse events may occur at a number of different points in the perioperative period (Box 5.2). Important preoperative risk factors generally relate to preexisting medical disease, whilst intraoperative risk factors may be associated with choice of anaesthetic, site of surgery or duration of procedure. In the postoperative period, adequacy of pain relief, anaemia, and oxygen therapy may be of importance. From the available data a relative risk-scoring system can be developed. This is then applied prospectively to a similar group of patients in order to validate the system. Examples of scoring systems and their usefulness will be reviewed later in this chapter.

Such scoring systems are, however, not perfect. They may, for example, only reflect the practice of a single institution. Conclusions drawn may be based on historical surgical or anaesthetic practices, no longer applicable. Many can only take into account the preoperative condition of the patient

Box 5.2 Risk factors associated with adverse events in the perioperative period

---

Preoperative risk factors
Preexisting medical disease
Age

Intraoperative risk factors
Emergency status
Type of anaesthetic
Nature and site of surgery
Duration of procedure
Haemodynamic stability
Monitoring
Experience of anaesthetist/surgeon/assistants

Postoperative risk factors
Availability of high-dependency care facility
Oxygen therapy
Pain relief
Anaemia

---

and will be unable to account for the effects of other perioperative events such as the nature of the intended surgery. It is therefore imperative when using these systems to be mindful of their innate faults.

Decide who might be harmed

The anaesthetist in his or her preoperative assessment of the patient assesses risk by drawing together information from the history and examination of the patient. This, coupled with the results of appropriate preoperative investigations, allows a patient risk profile to be established. Superimposed upon this will be the nature and complexity of the intended surgery and associated anaesthetic and postoperative management.

Evaluate the risks

This is the process whereby the anaesthetist assimilates the information gleaned from assessment of the patient and compares their given patient against a historical data set, either from published data or from their own experience and from management of similar patients over time. Following this process, the decision to proceed can be taken or further preoperative treatments and investigations instituted to optimise the condition of the patient in an attempt to lower the risks. If no further preoperative investigations or treatments are required or if delaying surgery will be associated with an increased risk to the patient, then the anaesthetist must decide the most appropriate anaesthetic management. Included in this decision will be a requirement to consider who should be managing the case from both surgical and anaesthetic perspectives and also the time of day that the surgery is scheduled. For example, evidence from the 1995–6 NCEPOD report suggests that "out of hours" operating is associated with a higher mortality.[4]

Record findings

It is essential that the preoperative assessment of a patient is recorded in the case notes, including recommendations for further investigation and treatment. Current practice in the UK health service can sometimes result in a patient being assessed by one anaesthetist and subsequently being administered anaesthesia by another anaesthetist.

Mathematical modelling

Risk assessment is a process which lends itself to mathematical modelling in order to predict outcome. Outcome in such circumstances can be defined as the condition of the patient following a given intervention. Any

81

patient variable used in the prediction of outcome is an *explanator*. In mathematical terms, outcome and explanator variables can be continuous, ordinal or categorical and must have easily reproducible and measurable endpoints. The construction of a predictive model in biological systems usually involves analysis of the effects of a number of explanator variables on a single outcome. This is known as multivariate analysis. It is important to ascertain whether explanator variables are independent or correlated; for example, start time of anaesthesia and knife to skin are correlated variables whilst start time of anaesthesia and length of hospital stay are not. Following validation of the acquired data, an appropriate model can be constructed.

Types of mathematical model

Multiple regression
This is a simple model in which independent weighting is given to an explanator variable and the overall outcome equates to the sum of the individual risk factors. Although a common model in use in non-biological systems, multiple regression analysis is not easily applied to risk assessment. The reasons for this are twofold. First, multiple regression can only be used in situations where an outcome variable is continuous and has a normal distribution of values, e.g. length of hospital stay. Second, explanator variables should have a multivariate normal distribution. This is often not the case in clinical practice.

Multiple logistic regression
A common model for risk assessment. Multiple logistic regression relies on the fact that in the majority of cases the outcome variable is a binary derivative, i.e. choice of x or y. This removes any requirement on the explanator variables to be normally distributed or of the same type. Multiple logistic regression models provide a predictive outcome probability that a patient will be in a defined group; common examples include risk of death or morbidity.

Bayesian model
Use of the Bayes' theorem is increasingly popular in the science of risk assessment. Described in 1763, Bayes' theorem or rule established a mathematical basis for probability inference, a mechanism by which the probability of an event occurring in the future is calculated from the number of times it has not occurred in the past. An established data set is used to form a probability matrix of explanator variables against outcome variables. It is an essential requirement that all the data variables are categorical. The advantage of the Bayesian model is that the data set can be constantly revised over time.

Indicators of risk

The anaesthetic literature contains numerous examples of preoperative risk assessment protocols. They range from simple severity of illness classifications, such as that described by the American Society of Anesthesiologists (ASA),[5] to complex weighted scoring systems which may be system or specialty specific; for example, the Goldman Cardiac Risk Index[6] and the Parsonnet Risk Index[7] used for patients with cardiac disease. There is, however, no simple way of assessing risk, in particular risk of morbidity, and no unifying system which can account for every eventuality. In addition, the acceptable level of risk may be altered depending on circumstances.

Severity of illness classifications

ASA classification of Physical Status

Originally commissioned in 1941 by the ASA, this was the first attempt to identify perioperative risk by the preoperative evaluation of a patient's physical status. The initial classification of four groups was extended to five in 1961 and the added risk of emergency procedures was identified by the addition of the letter "E" to the classification (Box 5.3). The system was officially adopted by the ASA in 1963, since when it has gained worldwide acceptance as a simple means of categorising patients presenting for surgery and anaesthesia. Based on the preoperative history and examination of the patient coupled with the results of any relevant investigations, the anaesthetist assigns the patient to one of five categories.

Its detractors feel that it is far too subjective, that it is not applicable to all patients (thus neonates and pregnant mothers are not easily classified) and that it does not take into account the nature of the intended surgery. It also fails to give weight to situations where patients present with systemic disease in more than one system and where there may be associated co-morbidity

---

Box 5.3 ASA classification of Physical Status

ASA 1 Normal healthy patient; no known organic, biochemical or psychiatric disease

ASA 2 Patient with mild-to-moderate systemic disease, e.g. mild asthmatic

ASA 3 Patient with severe systemic disease that limits normal activity, e.g. severe rheumatoid arthritis.

ASA 4 Patient with severe systemic disease that is a constant threat to life, e.g. unstable angina.

ASA 5 Patient who is moribund and unlikely to survive 24 hours whether operated upon or not

The addition of the letter "E" indicates those patients in whom emergency surgery is undertaken.

(for example, cardiorespiratory disease) or where patients without physical disease may be at increased risk (for example, anticipated difficult intubation, obesity, and the elderly).

The inherent subjectivity of the ASA classification has led to a plethora of alternative and potentially more objective scoring systems. These are either systems based, for example the Goldman Cardiac Risk Index for patients with cardiac disease, or based on patient physical status and operative procedure, for example the Parsonnet Risk Index for cardiac surgery. This quest for greater objectivity does, however, bring its own problems.

Systems-based risk assessment

Systems-based risk assessment is self-explanatory. The construction of a risk index requires a large database of patients and a good understanding of statistics and probability in order to ensure that the correct weighting is given to the various components of the scoring system. Appraisal of the literature shows that cardiac history and cardiac events related to pathophysiological changes in cardiac function and pulmonary disease associated with adverse changes in pulmonary function are the two main risk factors for untoward or adverse outcomes during the perioperative period. The drive for development of risk-adjusted outcome data has largely been in the field of cardiopulmonary disease.

Cardiac risk indices

The existence of cardiac disease in a patient presenting for non-cardiac surgery presents a considerable risk of both mortality and morbidity.[8] The majority of these events, however, take place in the postoperative period.[9] The most widely quoted risk index for patients with cardiac disease is that described by Goldman in 1977 (Table 5.1). This was the first real attempt to analyse risk of perioperative morbid events in a group of 1000 patients with preexisting cardiac disease.

Table 5.1 Preoperative factors relating to the development of postoperative cardiac complications[6]

Factor	Points
Gallop rhythm or elevated jugular venous pressure	11
Myocardial infarction in preceding six months	10
Rhythm other than sinus or premature atrial contractions on preoperative electrocardiogram	7
> 5 ventricular premature beats (VPBs) per minute	7
Age > 70 years	5
Emergency surgery	4
Intraperitoneal, intrathoracic or aortic operation	3
Poor general physical status	3
Significant aortic stenosis	3
Total possible points	53

The number of points which an individual patient accrues places them into one of four classes associated with an increasing risk of perioperative cardiac morbidity (Box 5.4). This risk index has been widely validated in large populations of patients undergoing various types of non-cardiac surgery. Concerns over its application to patients undergoing vascular surgery led to it being modified (Table 5.2).[10]

The American College of Physicians guidelines incorporate aspects of this revised classification into an algorithm for the perioperative management of patients with coronary artery disease undergoing non-cardiac vascular surgery.[11] Evidence supports the notion that patients with a score greater than 16 should undergo further diagnostic testing, especially if major vascular surgery is contemplated.

Major changes in management strategies for the treatment of acute myocardial infarction, including the use of thrombolytic agents, percutaneous transluminal angioplasty and coronary artery stenting, have altered,

Box 5.4 Classification of risk based on points scored in the Goldman Cardiac Risk Index[6]

Class 1	0–5 points
Class 2	6–12 points
Class 3	13–25 points
Class 4	>25 points

Table 5.2 Detsky modification of the Goldman Cardiac Risk Index[10]

Variables		Points
Angina		
	Class IV	20
	Class III	10
	Unstable angina <3 months	10
Suspected critical aortic stenosis		20
Myocardial infarction		
	< 6 months	10
	> 6 months	5
Pulmonary oedema		
	< 1 week	10
	Ever	5
Emergency surgery		10
Non-sinus rhythm		5
>5 ventricular premature beats		5
Poor general health		5
Age >70 years		5
Class I	Low risk	0–15
Class II	Intermediate risk	20–30
Class III	High risk	>30

and continue to alter the risk profile of patients presenting for non-cardiac surgery.

Cardiac risk and surgical procedure. As mentioned previously, the nature of the intended surgery can adversely affect outcome. There is little in the literature which helps to define surgery-specific related cardiac complications. One study utilising data from the Coronary Artery Surgery Study (CASS) has achieved this.[12] In a retrospective analysis of patients with known cardiac disease randomised to medical treatment or coronary artery bypass prior to non-cardiac surgery, the incidence of perioperative cardiac events and their relationship to the type of surgery were noted. The findings are summarised in Box 5.5. Cardiac risk indices continue to be modified and updated in the light of changing therapies and advances in the management of cardiac disease coupled with evidence-based evaluation of risk strategies.

Pulmonary risk indices

Pulmonary complications are frequent causes of perioperative morbidity and mortality in all types of surgery.[13] Chronic lung disease, frequently caused by cigarette smoking, is common in the hospital population and in order to reduce the incidence of perioperative respiratory complications, it is essential to have a framework for risk assessment. Attempts to produce a unified approach to pulmonary risk have been largely unsuccessful.

A number of studies utilising history and clinical examination have identified patients at risk of pulmonary complications. In the same studies, however, preoperative pulmonary function tests were not identified as being

---

Box 5.5 Cardiac risk stratification related to non-cardiac procedures[12]

Low risk: <1% chance of death or non-fatal myocardial infarction
- Endoscopic surgery
- Peripheral surgery
- Ocular surgery
- Breast surgery

Intermediate risk: 1–5% chance of death or non-fatal myocardial infarction
- Carotid artery surgery
- Major head and neck surgery
- Elective intraabdominal or intrathoracic surgery
- Orthopaedic procedures
- Prostatic surgery

High risk: >5% chance of death or non-fatal myocardial infarction
- Emergency operations, especially in the elderly
- Major vascular surgery
- Peripheral vascular surgery
- Procedures associated with massive blood loss or fluid shifts

discriminatory independent risk factors.[13-16] This inability to predict accurate perioperative morbidity for patients with respiratory disease is indicative of the high incidence of co-morbidity in this group of patients. In one study looking at patients undergoing abdominal surgery, 33% had both cardiac and pulmonary complications postoperatively.[17] In such circumstances it is impossible to attribute the risk due to pulmonary disease independently and overall risk can only be assessed using a multifactorial scoring system. An example of such a multifactorial scoring system has been developed for patients undergoing lung resection.[18] The Cardiopulmonary Risk Index (CPRI) is a combination of the Goldman Cardiac Risk Index value (scored from 1 to 4), plus a pulmonary risk index (scored from 1 to 6), based on the presence of any of the factors listed in Box 5.6. A combined total score of >4 is highly predictive of postoperative complications. In a subsequent study preoperative exercise testing was able to further define patient risk.[19] Critics of this system point out the highly subjective assessment of cough and wheeze and that the nature of intended surgery is not taken into account.[20]

A more objective approach to the assessment of postoperative risk of morbidity in patients undergoing lung resection, based on the calculation of a predictive respiratory complication quotient (PRQ), has been reported.[21] PRQ is calculated using a complex mathematical formula from the results of patient spirometry, carbon monoxide diffusion capacity, split lung function testing and an analysis of the effects of exercise on blood gases. A PRQ of less than 2200 was found to be associated with an increased risk of pulmonary complication. Whether such a system can be applied to predict respiratory complications in patients undergoing non-thoracic surgery has yet to be evaluated.

Attempts at risk assessment in patients with non-cardiopulmonary disease or in particular patient subgroups (the obstetric patient, children, etc.) or in association with a particular type of surgery (for example, urology or orthopaedic surgery) have not been successful nor found widespread

Box 5.6 Pulmonary risk index[18]

Obesity
Recent history of cigarette smoking
Cough
Diffuse wheeze
Elevated P_aCO_2 >6 kPa
FEV_1/FVC ratio <70% predicted

FEV_1, forced expiratory volume in one second; FVC, forced vital capacity
Presence of any factor scores 1 point. Maximum score 6 points

acceptance. This lack of success is largely related to the fact that the majority of perioperative-related adverse events are associated with preexisting cardiac or respiratory disease states. Where death or morbidity occur in patients without either of these, preoperative assessment does not reliably help to predict an adverse perioperative event.

Conclusion

Risk assessment is an important part of health-care management. There is increasing pressure on doctors from government and the public to supply data on risk-adjusted outcomes as a marker of quality of health care. For the individual anaesthetist there is a requirement to provide the patient with an evidence-based value for risk of a poor outcome associated with a given operative procedure. In the future doctors will be required to demonstrate that the risk to the patient for a given procedure as performed by them is comparable to that of their peers.

1 AAGBI. *Risk management*. London: Association of Anaesthetists of Great Britain and Ireland, 1998.
2 Warner MA, Shields SE, Shute CG *et al.* Major morbidity and mortality within 1 month of ambulatory surgery and anesthesia. *JAMA* 1993; 270: 1437–41.
3 HSE. *An introduction to health and safety*. London: HMSO, 1997.
4 *Who operates when?* London: NCEPOD, 1997.
5 American Society of Anesthesiologists. New classification of physical status. *Anesthesiology* 1963; 24: III.
6 Goldman L, Caldera D, Nussbaum SR *et al.* Multifactorial index of cardiac risk in non-cardiac surgical procedures. *N Engl J Med* 1977; 297: 845–50.
7 Parsonnet V, Dean D, Bernstein AD. A method of uniform stratification of risk for evaluating the results of surgery in acquired adult heart disease. *Circulation* 1989; 79: I3–I12.
8 Mangano DT. Perioperative cardiac morbidity. *Anesthesiology* 1990; 72: 153–84.
9 Coriat P. Reducing cardiovascular risk in patients undergoing non-cardiac surgery. *Curr Opin Anaesthesiol* 1998; 11: 311–14.
10 Detsky A, Abrams H, McLaughlin J *et al.* Predicting cardiac complications in patients undergoing non-cardiac surgery. *J Gen Intern Med* 1988; 1: 211–19.
11 Palda VA, Detsky AS. Perioperative assessment and management of risk from coronary artery disease. *Ann Intern Med* 1997; 127: 313–28.
12 Eagle KA, Rihal CS, Mickel MC *et al.* Cardiac risk and non-cardiac surgery: influence of coronary disease and type of surgery in 3368 operations. CASS investigators and University of Michigan Heart Care program. Coronary Artery Surgery Study. *Circulation* 1997; 96: 1882–7.
13 Mitchell CK, Smoger SH, Pfeifer MP *et al.* Multivariate analysis of factors associated with postoperative pulmonary complications following general elective surgery. *Arch Surg* 1998; 133: 194–8.
14 Blumam LG, Mosca L, Newman N *et al.* Preoperative smoking habits and pulmonary complications. *Chest* 1998; 113: 883–9.
15 Brooks-Brunn JA. Predictors of postoperative pulmonary complications following abdominal surgery. *Chest* 1997; 111: 564–71.
16 Wong DH, Weber EC, Schell MJ *et al.* Factors associated with postoperative pulmonary complications in patients with severe chronic obstructive pulmonary disease. *Anesth Analg* 1995; 80: 276–84.
17 Lawrence VA, Dhanda R, Hilsenbank SG *et al.* Risk of pulmonary complications after elective abdominal surgery. *Chest* 1996; 110: 744–50.

18 Epstein SK, Faling LJ, Daly BD *et al*. Predicting complications after pulmonary resection: preoperative exercise testing vs a multifactorial cardiopulmonary index. *Chest* 1993; **104**: 694–700.

19 Epstein SK, Faling LJ, Daly BD *et al*. Inability to perform bicycle ergometry predicts increased morbidity and mortality after lung resection. *Chest* 1995; **107**: 311–16.

20 Melendez JA, Carlon VA. Cardiopulmonary risk index does not predict complications after thoracic surgery. *Chest* 1998; **114**: 69–75.

21 Melendez JA, Barra R. Predictive respiratory complication quotient predicts pulmonary complications in thoracic surgical patients. *Ann Thorac Surg* 1998; **66**: 220–4.

SECTION 3: Preoperative preparation of the patient

6: Preoperative optimisation

VERGHESE T CHERIAN, ANDREW A TOMLINSON

Introduction

An increasing number of patients with significant co-morbidity present for anaesthesia and surgery. This is, at least in part, a consequence of the ageing population as well as the fact that modern anaesthesia is, in general, very safe. It is important to identify such patients so that an early preoperative assessment can be undertaken. At the initial visit, the "functional impairment" (the ability, or otherwise, to perform activities of daily living) caused by the disease process is assessed by the traditional approach of history, physical examination, and review of investigations. Indeed, at this visit the question must be asked as to whether or not the anticipated benefits of the proposed surgery are greater than the associated risks of anaesthesia and surgery. If the answer is yes, the clinician has to determine if the patient is in the optimum condition.

Preoperative optimisation involves, first, identifying that a patient's physical status can be improved and, second, implementing appropriate treatment regimens, amending current medication or both. Drug therapy will be the principal method used in most patients. However, physical therapies may also have an important role to play. The extent to which this occurs will depend upon the perceived urgency of the surgery. It is only recently that controlled studies have been undertaken to assess whether or not preoperative optimisation of the patient's physical condition results in lower morbidity. These studies appear to confirm a long-held view that such preoperative optimisation does lead to a lower perioperative morbidity and mortality, at least in patients with known disease of the cardiovascular system.[1-3]

It is important to remember that there is a continuum of medical care associated with surgery and clinicians in the different disciplines must work together to ensure that the best outcome occurs for individual patients. To this end, compromises have to be made as to how long surgery can be delayed to allow optimisation to occur. On occasion immediate surgery has to be performed, as any delay will result in death. In such cases the aim will

93

be to maintain the physiological status of the patient as near to the presumed normal as possible. Postponement of surgery for 2–4 hours often allows treatment to be started. Best of all is the surgical condition that can be delayed until optimal therapy has not only been started but given time to produce maximum benefit. This may put pressure on scarce resources such as high-dependency facilities if, for example, intensive preoperative cardiovascular optimisation is considered appropriate.

This chapter identifies common disease processes that are amenable to optimisation prior to surgery, given time and resources, and considers individual diseases under the appropriate systems.

Cardiovascular disease

Cardiovascular disease is common amongst patients presenting for anaesthesia and surgery and its prevalence increases with age. The most significant perioperative risk factors associated with adverse outcome have been identified as congestive heart failure (CHF), myocardial infarction (MI) within six months, unstable angina, significant arrhythmias, and severe valvular disease.[4,5] In addition to these major risk factors, the American College of Cardiology Task Force identified further, less significant clinical predictors of increased perioperative cardiovascular risk (Box 6.1).[5] Preoperative evaluation of individual patients' functional capacity should identify factors that are amenable to modification by further therapeutic interventions preoperatively.

Coronary artery disease

Coronary artery disease (CAD) is increasingly common in the ageing population and patients with easily induced ischaemia have an increased incidence of morbidity and mortality during the perioperative period. A careful history, physical examination, and electrocardiogram (ECG) assessment are essential to ensure that the presence of CAD is identified, as well as to assess its severity, stability, and efficacy of current treatment. In patients with known or suspected severe disease, the extent of affected myocardium, the degree of stress required to induce ischaemia and the ventricular function should be assessed further, using exercise thallium imaging, ECG-monitored exercise testing and echocardiography, respectively.

The extent of preoperative optimisation of a patient with CAD will be influenced by the urgency of surgery. Unfortunately, most surgical emergencies, such as major trauma and symptomatic abdominal aortic aneurysm, do not permit more than a cursory cardiac evaluation. In such situations, efforts should be made to maintain haemodynamic stability perioperatively using invasive monitoring and early surgery is essential to control bleeding. Whilst awaiting surgery, treatment to maintain arterial blood pressures that

Box 6.1 Predictors of increased perioperative cardiovascular morbidity (myocardial infarction, congestive heart failure) and mortality (reproduced with permission from reference[5])

Major
- Unstable coronary syndromes:
  recent myocardial infarction, unstable angina
- Decompensated congestive cardiac failure
- Significant arrhythmia:
  high-grade atrioventricular block
  symptomatic ventricular arrhythmias
  supraventricular arrhythmias with uncontrolled ventricular rate
- Severe valvular disease

Intermediate
- Mild angina pectoris
- Previous myocardial infarction by history or pathological Q waves
- Compensated congestive cardiac failure
- Diabetes mellitus

Minor
- Advanced age
- Abnormal ECG:
  left ventricular hypertrophy
  left bundle branch block
  ST segment abnormalities
- Rhythm other than sinus (e.g. atrial fibrillation)
- Low functional capacity (inability to climb one flight of stairs)
- History of stroke
- Uncontrolled hypertension

ensure adequate major organ perfusion should be instituted; this is particularly important in patients with a history of previous MI, as hypotension is associated with an increased incidence of reinfarction.[6] Such patients are especially challenging since the risk of further active bleeding from the primary surgical lesion increases as the blood pressure rises.

If surgery is not urgent and the patient is to benefit from it, factors that can be improved must be identified and further treatment instituted in the available time. Determining the patient's exercise tolerance gives an estimate of the dynamic status of the coronary circulation and the myocardium. In the absence of a recent exercise ECG, the functional capacity of the patient is assessed by their ability to perform activities of daily living.[5] The invasive investigation of coronary angiography is only indicated if the patient is a candidate for myocardial revascularisation; this includes patients who develop ischaemia at low levels of exercise and those with severe unstable angina. If the patient has undergone coronary revascularisation in the last five years or extensive coronary evaluation in the past two years and the clinical status remains stable, further cardiac evaluation is not necessary.[5]

Surgery-specific cardiac risk is related to the type of surgery and the associated haemodynamic stress.[5] Major surgical procedures, including intraabdominal and intrathoracic surgery, have been shown to increase perioperative ischaemia more than peripheral surgery.[7] Although these factors cannot be modified, they may influence the decision as to whether alternative, less invasive surgical, or non-surgical, treatment is preferable.

Patients with a proven myocardial infarction in the previous six months
A history of previous MI significantly increases the risk of reinfarction and, historically, elective surgery was postponed for six months. It has been suggested that the advent of thrombolytic therapy for the treatment of acute MI now makes it reasonable to consider reducing the delay to 4–6 weeks post-MI for elective surgery.[7] Patients with a recent MI should be assessed for ongoing risk of myocardial ischaemia. Individuals who survive a non-Q wave infarction are at greater risk of reinfarction and efforts should be made to maintain good oxygen supply while reducing oxygen demand, whilst those who survive a Q wave (transmural) infarction are at increased risk of developing arrhythmias.[7]

The use of invasive monitoring and the rapid treatment of fluctuations in cardiovascular variables has been shown to reduce perioperative reinfarction.[7] In addition, the pharmacological optimisation of left ventricular function and oxygen transport with the aid of pulmonary artery floatation catheters in an intensive care unit appears to reduce perioperative cardiac morbidity.[1,3] Such management should be considered for any patient with a history of severe CAD (including those with severe unstable angina) who requires surgery that is likely to increase perioperative ischaemia.

Myocardial oxygen supply is dependent upon the maintenance of an adequate diastolic blood pressure, haemoglobin concentration, and oxygen saturation. These factors must be optimised. Myocardial oxygen demand can be minimised by the use of β-blockers, which help to obtund the inotropic and chronotropic effects of excessive sympathetic stimulation. The perioperative administration of intravenous atenolol significantly reduces heart rate as well as the incidence of postoperative myocardial ischaemia.[2] Vasodilators such as nitroglycerine reduce myocardial oxygen demand by reducing afterload, thereby decreasing ventricular wall tension, which may be beneficial. When reducing the left ventricular work, it is important to ensure that adequate perfusion is maintained to other organs to prevent organ failure. Thus the overall strategy is one of minimising cardiac work, whilst augmenting oxygen delivery to the heart and other organs.

Rarely, coronary artery bypass graft (CABG) surgery may be indicated before non-cardiac surgery if the stress of such surgery is considered to exceed the stress of daily life and the non-cardiac surgical procedure is associated with a good outcome.[5]

Patients with angina

Although many patients with CAD presenting for surgery will be taking β-blockers, the dose is often suboptimal (usually because of concerns over bradycardia during daily living) and therefore there may be an opportunity to intensify treatment.[8] Other antianginal therapy should be optimised and elective surgery delayed, if necessary, to allow this to be accomplished. All such medication must be continued through to the morning of surgery. Patients with unstable angina are known to have an increased perioperative risk and those undergoing surgery associated with an increased risk of perioperative ischaemia should be considered for intensive perioperative monitoring, as previously discussed.

Hypercoagulability, which encourages microthrombi formation in the coronary arteries and intramyocardial arterioles, is another recognised cause of acute postoperative myocardial ischaemia. Aspirin, by virtue of its antiplatelet action, plays a major role in the primary and secondary prevention of myocardial ischaemia and its use may be of benefit perioperatively in patients with known CAD,[8] although the increased risks of intraoperative bleeding must be considered.

In patients with intermediate cardiovascular risk factors such as MI more than six months ago and diabetes mellitus, consideration of the functional capacity of the patient and type of surgery allows a rational approach to identifying which patients may benefit from further investigations. Patients with moderate-to-excellent functional capacity can normally undergo surgery with little likelihood of perioperative cardiac morbidity, as can patients with minor clinical predictors and moderate-to-excellent functional capacity.[5]

Congestive heart failure

Heart failure is a common disease for which hospital admissions are rising rapidly.[9] Patients with severe congestive heart failure (CHF) have an unacceptably high incidence of perioperative mortality and surgery should be deferred for all but immediate life-saving procedures.[4,5] This serious disturbance of myocardial function results from direct myocardial damage (for example, MI, cardiomyopathy) or chronic exposure of the myocardium to excessive haemodynamic workload (such as hypertension, valvular heart disease).

The immediate management is directed towards increasing myocardial oxygen supply (oxygen therapy, maintaining diastolic blood pressure and promoting coronary vasodilatation) and reducing its oxygen demand (reducing tachycardia and afterload, maintaining adequate preload and minimising arrhythmias). Management of CHF should be in consultation with the cardiology team and, ideally, should be undertaken in an intensive care unit using invasive monitoring to help titrate therapy. Medical management of CHF has focused on bedrest, oxygen therapy, intravenous diuretic therapy, treatment of severe hypertension and cardiac arrhythmias, and intravenous diamorphine. Angiotensin-converting enzyme (ACE) inhibitors are helpful in optimising cardiac function in CHF but should be started at low doses to avoid sudden hypotension. The use of β-blockers in conjunction with ACE inhibitors has been shown to reduce the mortality from this condition, although their use should be overseen by a cardiologist, at least in the first instance.[9] In severe CHF, with a systolic blood pressure above 100 mmHg, a low-dose infusion of glyceryltrinitrate helps reduce left ventricular afterload. Use of an inodilator (for example, dobutamine or dopexamine) has the advantage of improving cardiac output while reducing afterload.

Cardiac arrhythmias

Cardiac arrhythmias and conduction disturbances are common findings in the perioperative period. Both supraventricular and ventricular arrhythmias have been identified as independent risk factors for perioperative cardiac morbidity, as they may reflect underlying serious cardiopulmonary disease, drug toxicity or metabolic derangement. Although rare, arrhythmias may deteriorate into life-threatening rhythm disturbances because of the haemodynamic or metabolic derangement they cause. Any underlying cause should be corrected if possible, before therapy is initiated for symptomatic or haemodynamically significant arrhythmia. The indications for antiarrhythmic therapy and cardiac pacing are identical to the non-operative setting.[5] Although the following provides information on the initial management of the most common arrhythmias,[10] a detailed discussion of all arrhythmias is beyond the scope of this chapter. It is prudent to seek the advice of a cardiologist, as the diagnosis of the exact arrhythmia can be challenging.

Bradyarrhythmias

Bradycardia is defined as a heart rate of less than 60 beats per minute. However, not all patients with rates below this require treatment, the deciding factor being the patient's haemodynamic state. The decision to treat will depend upon the clinical signs and whether the rhythm has the potential to proceed to asystole.

Sinus bradycardia. Even in the fit patient, a heart rate below 40 per minute is often poorly tolerated and should be treated if hypotension, ventricular arrhythmia or signs of poor peripheral perfusion are observed in the perioperative period. Treatment should commence with intravenous atropine and continue through ephedrine, adrenaline (epinephrine) or isoprenaline (isoproterenol) to transvenous pacing, if drug therapy fails.

Sinus node dysfunction. Sinus node dysfunction with associated symptoms of conduction disturbance requires the insertion of a pacemaker preoperatively.

Atrioventricular (AV) conduction defects. First-degree AV block and Mobitz type 1 second-degree block (disease of the AV node) are relatively benign and do not require treatment. Mobitz type 2 second-degree block (disease of the bundle of His) may progress to complete heart block and thus requires insertion of a pacemaker prior to major surgery. Patients with symptomatic third-degree block should also have a pacemaker inserted preoperatively, if not already present.

Interventricular conduction defects. Many patients with such disease do not require active treatment. Those with sudden onset bifascicular block (right bundle branch block and left axis deviation), alternating left and right bundle branch block, bifascicular block with unexplained syncope or non-drug induced trifascicular block require transvenous pacing preoperatively, as all are associated with an increased risk of asystole.

Permanent pacemakers. Permanent pacemakers must be checked preoperatively to verify normal function, as well as to identify the patient's level of pacemaker dependency. In pacemaker-dependent patients, electrocautery poses a special problem and appropriate measures must be instituted. The possibility of converting the pacemaker to fixed mode preoperatively should be considered on the advice of a cardiologist. Finally, serum potassium levels must be maintained within normal limits.

Tachyarrhythmias
Sinus tachycardia. Sinus tachycardia is usually physiological and the cause should be identified and treated (for example, blood loss, heart failure, thyrotoxicosis). If there is no obvious cause and it is causing significant haemodynamic compromise, the use of atenolol should be considered.

Broad-complex tachycardias. Broad-complex tachycardias should be considered ventricular until proved otherwise and the urgency of treatment will depend upon the clinical state. Treatment of the asymptomatic patient consists of correcting hypokalaemia and abnormalities of other electrolytes (including magnesium) and intravenous lignocaine. If this treatment is ineffective or the patient is haemodynamically compromised, synchronised cardioversion may be required. Intravenous amiodarone is an alternative treatment option in the asymptomatic patient.

Narrow-complex tachycardias. Narrow-complex tachycardias originate from the sinus node, atrium or AV junction and are less frequent and less hazardous to patients than ventricular tachycardia. Occasionally the arrhythmia may be atrial fibrillation, which can be difficult to diagnose at fast rates. Initial treatment consists of vagal stimulation by carotid sinus massage or a valsalva manoeuvre. In the haemodynamically stable patient, intravenous adenosine is the next treatment of choice (beware unpleasant side effects) followed by intravenous amiodarone. For the severely compromised patient, immediate cardioversion is required. If this is unsuccessful, it may need to be repeated after pretreatment with intravenous amiodarone.

Atrial fibrillation (AF). Chronic AF is the most common arrhythmia seen in clinical practice. The loss of atrial systolic function can reduce cardiac output by up to 50%, especially in those with coincident ventricular impairment.[11] In addition, patients are at increased risk of thromboembolism. The restoration and maintenance of sinus rhythm by electrical or chemical cardioversion is therefore desirable. Cardioversion is safe and most effective when delivered soon after the onset of AF. Restoration and maintenance of sinus rhythm after successful cardioversion may be enhanced by the use of antiarrhythmic therapy. Several drugs that affect atrial electrophysiology can terminate AF. These include flecainide, procainamide, and amiodarone although optimal therapy has yet to be determined.[12] Patients who are unstable will require immediate cardioversion. Control of the ventricular rate is sometimes necessary and in patients without ventricular preexcitation, this is most effective with intravenous verapamil, diltiazem or β-blockers.[12] β-blockers are especially effective in the presence of thyrotoxicosis. Digoxin should be considered as first-line treatment in patients with AF and congestive heart failure.

In patients with chronic AF, the risk of thromboembolism is significant and this can be reduced by the use of warfarin, although its use is not without risk if the international normalised ratio (INR) is maintained above the range 1.5–3.0.[11] Surgery is best delayed until the INR is 1.5 or less.

Ventricular arrhythmias
Premature ventricular contractions, complex ventricular ectopy, and non-sustained ventricular tachycardia usually do not require treatment except in the presence of ongoing or threatened myocardial ischaemia or moderate-to-severe left ventricular dysfunction.[5] Treatment options will depend upon the patient's ability to tolerate the haemodynamic disturbance. The degree of haemodynamic instability will determine whether immediate cardioversion or drug therapy is appropriate. A cardiology opinion is prudent in many instances. Premature ventricular contractions (PVCs) may indicate coronary artery disease, digoxin toxicity with hypokalaemia or hypoxia. PVCs may progress to ventricular tachycardia or fibrillation if they are multiple (more than five per minute), multifocal, bigeminal or near the vulnerable period of the preceding ventricular depolarisation (R-on-T). The first step is to correct underlying abnormalities. Active treatment is only

indicated if haemodynamic instability is evident, even with more than five PVCs per minute. Lignocaine, by slow intravenous injection, is the treatment of choice, followed by an infusion of lignocaine if the arrhythmia persists.

Valvular heart disease

Severe aortic stenosis poses a great risk for non-cardiac surgery and elective surgery should be postponed until aortic valve replacement or balloon valvoplasty has been undertaken.[5] Patients with mitral stenosis tolerate tachycardia (reduced diastolic filling time) and vasodilatation ("fixed" cardiac output) poorly. β-blockers and calcium channel blockers are effective in reducing the heart rate.

Premedication should be sufficient to allay anxiety, whilst avoiding oversedation. In patients with aortic regurgitation, careful attention to intravascular fluid volume and reduction of afterload is essential. Patients with severe mitral regurgitation also benefit from afterload reduction and the preoperative administration of diuretic therapy (although they are able to tolerate mildly increased heart rates). Good premedication in conjunction with calcium channel blockers reduces afterload. An understanding of the haemodynamics of the valvular lesion, optimisation of the ventricular preload and afterload, and antibiotics for endocarditis prophylaxis are all important aspects of the preoperative preparation of these patients.

Hypertension

Goldman and colleagues showed that *mild* (systolic blood pressure [SBP] 140–159 mmHg; diastolic blood pressure [DBP] 90–99 mmHg) to *moderate* (SBP 160–179 mmHg; DBP 100–109 mmHg) hypertension, even with inadequate control, need not subject patients to added risk provided they are closely monitored and treated to ensure both hypertensive and hypotensive episodes were avoided.[4,13] Exaggerated intraoperative blood pressure fluctuations with associated ECG evidence of myocardial ischaemia have been demonstrated in patients with *severe* hypertension (SBP 180–209 mmHg; DBP 110–119 mmHg).[14] It follows that, where possible, preoperative control of blood pressure in patients with severe hypertension is prudent.[5] β-blockers lead to effective modulation of blood pressure and the reduction in number and duration of perioperative ischaemic episodes[2] and, provided there are no contraindications, their use is recommended. The calcium channel blocker nifedipine is an alternative when β-blockers are contraindicated. The speed with which control is achieved can be tailored to the urgency of surgery although it must be remembered that sustained hypertension alters cerebral autoregulation and sudden reductions in pressure may reduce cerebral perfusion. Therefore the reduction of blood pressure should be controlled carefully and occur over a minimum of 12 hours.

If the initial evaluation establishes mild or moderate hypertension and there are no associated cardiovascular or metabolic abnormalities, there is no need to delay surgery. Any evidence of associated complications should delay surgery whilst appropriate treatment is instituted using current guidelines.[15] For the treated hypertensive, all medication should be continued until the day of surgery, with the exception of diuretics which may cause dehydration in a fasted patient, and ACE inhibitors which can cause marked hypotension in combination with the use of inhalational anaesthetic agents.[16] It is important to review the patient's baseline blood pressure measurements to assess control and aim to maintain the preoperative pressure intraoperatively. In the anxious patient with a sustained raised blood pressure, sedative premedication may lower the blood pressure, but it has no effect on the underlying cardiac disease.

Respiratory disease

The successful anaesthetic management of patients with respiratory disease depends upon an accurate assessment of the functional impairment caused by the disease process, as well as an appreciation of the effects of anaesthesia and surgery on the pulmonary function. Preoperative management must aim to optimise gas exchange and ensure that intra- and postoperative pulmonary complications are minimised.

Reactive airway disease

The term "reactive airway disease" is considered synonymous with asthma. Airway reactivity is also increased in patients with allergic rhinitis, bronchitis, emphysema, and respiratory viral infections. Whilst asthmatics have *chronic* hyperreactivity of their airways, patients with upper respiratory infections have *acute* airway reactivity, which may last for up to six weeks after the initial viral infection.[17]

Asthma

A practical classification for grading asthma based on history was suggested by Kingston and Hirschman (Table 6.1).[18]

When assessing an asthmatic patient for surgery, the importance of a detailed history, examination and use of simple spirometry testing cannot be overemphasised. The forced vital capacity (FVC), forced expiratory volume in 1 second (FEV_1), and the peak expiratory flow rate (PEFR) may be reduced and the percentage reduction in these parameters is used to

Table 6.1 Classification of asthma[18]

Group	History	Suggested intervention
I	Past history of wheezing Currently asymptomatic Not taking any medication	Routine physical examination Spirometry desirable
II	History of recurrent bronchospasm Currently not wheezing Taking regular medication	Routine physical examination Spirometry necessary Preoperative bronchodilators and corticosteroids
III	Active wheezing restricting daily activities Currently on high-dose medication	Spirometry necessary Blood gas analysis necessary Intensify therapy and defer elective surgery

grade the severity of the asthma. A reduction of 50% in the predicted value indicates severe impairment in pulmonary function. Hypercarbia and/or severe hypoxia is seen only in asthmatics with a FEV_1 of less than 25% or a PEFR of less than 30%. Postoperative mechanical ventilation may be indicated in these patients.

The mainstay of pharmacological preoperative preparation is the optimisation of bronchodilator therapy. In the past, the drug management of asthma focused on bronchial smooth muscle constriction and its reversibility. Current strategies for the management of asthma stress the importance of first switching off the inflammatory processes that trigger bronchoconstriction and mucosal oedema, by the early use of inhaled corticosteroids.[19] The drugs available to combat bronchospasm in asthmatic patients can therefore be divided into two major groups: antiinflammatory drugs and bronchodilators. Commonly, combinations of drugs are required to provide optimum treatment.

Antiinflammatory drugs
Glucocorticoids (GCS). Inhaled GCS are the most effective antiinflammatory agents available for treating asthma, although their onset of action is 6–12 hours.[19,20] Treatment with inhaled corticosteroid is optimised to the lowest effective maintenance dose by titrating the dose against symptoms and PEFR. The maximum effective daily dose of inhaled steroid for most adults is 800 μg. The potential for systemic adverse effects from higher doses usually outweighs any marginal therapeutic benefit and therefore a second-line drug (β_2-agonist, leukotriene antagonist) should be added if necessary. The possibility of adrenal suppression needs to be considered in patients on higher doses of inhaled steroid (above 800 mg daily in adults).[19,21]

Leukotriene antagonists. Leukotrienes are synthesised from arachidonic acid by 5-lipoxygenase and are important mediators for inflammation and smooth muscle constriction. Leukotriene antagonists, such as zafirlukast and montelukast, exhibit both bronchodilator and antiinflammatory activity and work within 24 hours.[19]

Bronchodilators
β_2-*adrenergic agonists*. These drugs act primarily on the bronchial smooth muscle, producing bronchodilatation. They are the first-line treatment for acute asthma (to buy time for the antiinflammatory effect of steroids to work) and are frequently used as second-line treatment in chronic asthma in combination with steroids. When administered by inhalation, the short acting β_2-agonists such as salbutamol and terbutaline have a maximal effect within 30 minutes and a duration of 4–6 hours. When patients present for surgery with an associated acute attack of asthma, nebulised salbutamol is the drug of choice, repeated every 30 minutes. There is some evidence that additional intravenous salbutamol improves the initial bronchodilator response obtained from the nebulised drug.[20] Patients taking regular β_2-agonists may require higher doses during an acute attack because of β_2-agonist induced downregulation of pulmonary β_2-adrenoreceptors. Corticosteroids have been shown to prevent this downregulation and therefore should be introduced in an acute episode, if not already part of a patient's treatment regimen.[20]

Theophylline. This drug increases the level of cAMP by inhibiting phosphodiesterase, resulting in smooth muscle relaxation. The bronchodilator action is weak but it does show some antiinflammatory effect. The main disadvantages are potential drug interactions, effects on metabolism, and low therapeutic index (therapeutic serum level is 10–20 µg/ml). As its bronchodilator response depends upon adequate blood concentrations which require monitoring, there is little place for its use in acute asthma, except in life-threatening emergencies when β_2-agonists have failed.

Other drugs
Anticholinergics. The rationale for the use of these drugs is the presence of increased airway vagal tone. The bronchodilating effect of these drugs is slow in onset and benefit has not been consistently demonstrated in asthmatic patients. In contrast, patients with chronic obstructive pulmonary disease may benefit from their use.[21]

Asthma therapy overview
In summary, for those patients presenting with mild-to-moderate symptoms of asthma, inhaled corticosteroids should be used as first-line antiinflammatory treatment although their onset of action is slow. A leukotriene antagonist may be added as second-line antiinflammatory therapy. Theophylline is a cheaper alternative for second-line therapy but has a lower therapeutic index. β_2-agonists remain the drugs of choice in

acute reversible bronchospasm and are highly effective in preventing bronchospasm when used shortly before exercise or exposure to known allergens or prior to endotracheal intubation. Regular medication should be continued, therefore, in all asthmatic patients and the preoperative addition of β_2-agonists is advisable in those whose symptoms are not controlled by corticosteroids.

For major surgery, pharmacological optimisation should occur in conjunction with routine chest physiotherapy and the bacteriological examination of sputum if present. This will help determine optimum antibiotic therapy in the event of postoperative chest infection, which is more prevalent in the asthmatic patient. Active infection must be treated preoperatively. In the presence of acute asthma, all but life-threatening emergency surgery should be postponed until the acute bronchospasm has been relieved and steroid therapy has been given time to work.

Upper respiratory tract infection

Airway reactivity is increased considerably during, and immediately after, upper respiratory tract infections. This hyperreactivity is neurally mediated and reflex vagal bronchoconstriction is enhanced. Children with upper respiratory tract infections are 2–7 times more likely to have adverse events in the perioperative period. If the child requires endotracheal intubation, the risk of respiratory complications increases 11-fold.[22] For all children (and probably adults), elective surgery that requires endotracheal intubation should be delayed for 4–6 weeks following a significant upper respiratory tract infection.

Chronic obstructive pulmonary disease

Chronic obstructive pulmonary disease (COPD) is characterised by airflow obstruction accompanied by features of chronic bronchitis, emphysema or both. It is a disease that characteristically affects middle-aged and elderly people and is one of the leading causes of morbidity and mortality worldwide.[23] The airflow obstruction in COPD is mostly irreversible and progressive, but is frequently accompanied by airway hyperreactivity. The airflow obstruction is not uniform throughout the lung and this contributes to ventilation-perfusion mismatch. Abnormal pulmonary gas exchange is a common feature of COPD and mismatching of ventilation and perfusion results in arterial hypoxaemia. Patients with COPD have a higher incidence of postoperative pulmonary complications such as bronchospasm, prolonged mechanical ventilation, and pneumonia. The preoperative optimisation of these patients is directed towards relieving any acute bronchospasm and treating specific abnormalities such as hypoxia, excessive bronchial secretions, and infection.

Pharmacological optimisation includes the use of β_2-agonists and anti-cholinergic agents. Both groups of drugs achieve short-term bronchodilatation and relieve symptoms in many people with COPD. There is evidence, however, that combining both groups provides better bronchodilatation than either drug alone[23] and combined optimal therapy is recommended. Inhaled corticosteroids may confer some long-term benefit in reducing exacerbations of moderate-to-severe COPD, but they do not provide short-term improvement.[23]

Other preoperative measures include chest physiotherapy and humidification of inspired gases to aid expectoration. The use of incentive spirometry in conjunction with physiotherapy may help reduce the incidence of postoperative pulmonary complications, although the evidence for this is conflicting. It is important to detect and treat any intercurrent infection with appropriate antibiotics, following Gram stain and culture of sputum. Finally, radiological examination is important to rule out spontaneous pneumothorax or emphysematous bullae.

Smoking

The clinical effects of cigarette smoking on the cardiovascular and respiratory systems are of great concern to the anaesthetist.[24] Smoking increases oxygen demand through nicotine activation of the sympathoadrenergic system, while decreasing oxygen carriage by raising carboxyhaemoglobin levels. Smoking is also a major risk for arterial thromboembolism and coronary vasospasm. Important respiratory system changes include mucus hypersecretion and impaired tracheobronchial clearance, as well as small airway narrowing with increased closing capacity, resulting in ventilation-perfusion mismatch. There is also increased airway reactivity. The terminal half-life of nicotine is two hours, although during regular smoking nicotine will accumulate and may persist overnight.[25] The half-life of carboxyhaemoglobin is four hours, but is prolonged by sleep.[25] Thus despite abstinence from smoking overnight, smokers may be exposed to the deleterious effects of nicotine and carboxyhaemoglobin on the cardiovascular system the next morning; this is most significant for patients with ischaemic heart disease. It is therefore preferable for patients to be "smoking free" for 24 hours preoperatively to gain significant cardiovascular benefit. The deleterious effects of smoking on pulmonary function take much longer to reverse; abstinence for six weeks is necessary to alter respiratory postoperative morbidity caused by smoking.

It is important that smokers stop smoking for as long as possible preoperatively. Although six weeks or more is the ideal this is frequently not possible given the addictive nature of smoking. It may be better, and more realistic, to try to persuade patients of the benefits of complete abstinence for the 24 hours prior to surgery. This is only possible in patients undergoing elective surgery and requires help from surgical colleagues and better patient education, although one attempt at this strategy was not particularly successful.[25]

Pneumothorax

Patients most at risk are those suffering recent trauma, those with asthma, and those with chronic lung disease with associated bullae. The presence of a pneumothorax should be ruled out before induction of general anaesthesia as it presents a considerable hazard. Intermittent positive pressure ventilation, the presence of coughing and straining and the use of nitrous oxide can all result in rapid increases in the size of the pneumothorax, with catastrophic results. The presence of a pneumothorax can be detected by clinical and radiological examination of the chest. If detected, a chest drain with an underwater seal should be inserted prior to the induction of general anaesthesia. A small (<30%) pneumothorax can be left untreated if surgery is to be undertaken using a local or regional technique, provided such a technique does not involve the risk of pneumothorax in the contralateral thoracic cavity!

Endocrine disease

The stress of surgery and anaesthesia produces marked endocrine changes affecting glucose and protein metabolism, fluid and electrolyte balance, and host defence mechanisms. Optimisation of preoperative treatments can help reduce associated fluctuations.

Diabetes mellitus

Diabetes mellitus is the most common endocrine disease encountered in anaesthetic practice. Generally, the preoperative anaesthetic management focuses on the prevention of extreme fluctuations in the blood glucose concentrations. It should also include an assessment of the presence of associated complications including CAD, hypertension, nephropathy, and neuropathy. End-organ complications related to diabetes are also important and there is an increasing awareness that the presence of autonomic neuropathy is associated with the possibility of sudden death syndrome in these patients.[26]

Autonomic neuropathy

The presence of autonomic neuropathy is associated with increased cardiovascular instability during anaesthesia, as homeostatic reflexes are unable to compensate for the effects of anaesthetic agents on vascular tone and myocardial contractility. This could be due to impaired catecholamine release.[27] Bradycardia and hypotension may not respond to the usual drug therapy (atropine and ephedrine) and may require the early administration of epinephrine.[27]

When reviewing a patient preoperatively, the presence of autonomic neuropathy can be assessed clinically by demonstrating a lack of pulse rate change on inspiration or orthostatic manoeuvres (standing up from the supine position). Review of the preoperative ECG may demonstrate the presence of decreased variability in the R-R interval as well as prolongation of the QT interval, both of which are suggestive of autonomic neuropathy. Adequate preoperative intravascular volume loading is important in patients with evidence of autonomic neuropathy (0.9% saline being the most appropriate solution), to help reduce the unwanted haemodynamic response to anaesthetic drugs.[27]

Metabolic control

Important points to consider when preparing a diabetic patient for surgery include the nature and urgency of surgery, the adequacy of blood glucose control, the treatment regimen used, and the anticipated time of return to a normal diet. The patient's record of blood and urine glucose testing and measurement of glycosylated haemoglobin (HbA1C) gives an estimate of long-term diabetic control. Diabetes may be type 1 (absolute insulin deficiency) or type 2 (compromised insulin secretion and insulin resistance).

The modern classification removes the term "non-insulin dependent diabetes" and with it the notion that such patients do not require insulin perioperatively. The need for insulin therapy must be guided by blood glucose levels. Patients with type 2 diabetes, managed with diet alone, need no specific intervention preoperatively. Patients on long-acting sulphonylureas (for example, chlorpropamide and glibenclamide) should, ideally, be switched to a drug with a shorter half-life three days preoperatively to prevent perioperative hypoglycaemia.[28] Unfortunately, this is frequently impractical and discontinuation 48 hours preoperatively is an acceptable alternative, albeit with less "tight" blood glucose control. The biguanide metformin may cause lactic acidosis when renal function is impaired and should be withdrawn 48–72 hours before surgery with, if possible, change to a short-acting sulphonylurea.[28] All oral hypoglycaemics should be omitted on the morning of surgery.

Patients who are found to be poorly controlled at preoperative assessment should be switched to an insulin regimen preoperatively and then treated as for a type 1 diabetic patient. Well-controlled type 1 diabetic patients managed on twice-daily regimens of short- and intermediate-acting insulin should continue with their regular medication until the morning of surgery, whilst those on a long-acting insulin should be converted to a short-acting insulin regimen three days preoperatively, if practical. In poorly controlled type 1 diabetic patients, elective surgery should be postponed until control is achieved with a short-acting insulin.

Types 1 and 2 diabetic patients requiring emergency or urgent surgery should have blood glucose levels monitored regularly and hypo- and hyperglycaemia managed appropriately with intravenous glucose and insulin.

There is no single protocol that can be used to manage all patients during the perioperative period. Ideally, the blood glucose should be maintained between 6 and 10 mmol/l; hypoglycaemia presents the greatest risk and it is safer to have slightly increased blood glucose levels. The variable stress responses to major surgery demand flexible insulin regimes. For patients undergoing intermediate and major surgery, this can be provided by a continuous infusion of glucose (with potassium added as necessary) and insulin. The insulin may be added directly to the glucose and potassium infusion or a continuous insulin infusion may be run through a separate pump via the same intravenous cannula as the glucose solution using a one-way valve.[29] With either method, the intravenous site should be checked frequently for signs of extravasation. For type 1 patients undergoing minor surgery, omission of the morning dose (and breakfast), monitoring of the blood glucose and early return to a normal diet with the usual insulin regime is all that is necessary. Whichever system is used, it is best commenced preoperatively and the key is to set clear goals and monitor blood glucose and serum potassium levels frequently.

Ketoacidosis
Poorly controlled diabetics may have significant metabolic decompensation, including ketoacidosis. Ketoacidotic patients are dehydrated (average deficit of 6 litres), potassium and sodium depleted and acidotic. The fluid and electrolyte disturbances are potentially life threatening and it is mandatory to correct them before surgery. Initial fluid replacement should consist of rapid infusion of 0.9% saline (approximately 3 litres in the first three hours). Insulin therapy must be commenced with frequent blood glucose monitoring as the glucose level may fall precipitously in the first two hours and an infusion of 5% dextrose commenced once the blood glucose falls to 13 mmol/l. Potassium must be replaced as its plasma concentration falls with the correction of the acidosis. Increased renal excretion of magnesium can occur in these patients with the possibility of associated cardiac arrhythmia. In ketoacidosis, plasma levels of ketone bodies are increased, contributing to an increased anion gap (greater than 16 mmol/l).

Management of these patients should be guided by frequent (initially half hourly) measurements of blood glucose, electrolytes, and pH. In the ketoacidotic diabetic patient all elective surgery must be deferred; however, it may be necessary to perform urgent operations, such as abscess drainage or amputation of a gangrenous limb, to remove the focus of infection and allow complete control to be achieved. Such surgery must only be undertaken once the dehydration has been corrected.

109

Thyroid disease

With the exception of diabetes and infertility, diseases of the thyroid are the most common endocrine disorders encountered clinically. They are more common in females than males. Thyroid hormones (T_3 and T_4) play a pivotal role in the control of metabolism, with excessive secretion (hyperthyroidism) leading to hypermetabolism and underactivity (hypothyroidism) leading to hypometabolism.

Hyperthyroidism

Clinical features of hyperthyroidism include weight loss, anxiety, muscle weakness, diarrhoea, menstrual abnormalities, intolerance to heat, tachycardia, cardiac arrhythmia, and heart failure. As a result, hyperthyroid patients who require surgical removal of the thyroid gland, or need surgery for unrelated reasons, should be rendered euthyroid preoperatively unless life-saving surgery is required.

Antithyroid drugs are used for the long-term treatment of hyperthyroidism as well as for the preoperative preparation of patients for thyroidectomy. Carbimazole and propylthiouracil act primarily by interfering with the synthesis of thyroid hormones. Carbimazole, 20–60 mg daily, is administered until the patient is euthyroid (4–6 weeks).[30] Potassium iodide is commenced 10 days preoperatively, to reduce both the concentration of circulating hormone and the vascularity of the thyroid gland. The β-adrenoceptor blocker propranolol (40–120 mg daily) blocks peripheral effects of the thyroid hormones and is used in conjunction with the antithyroid drugs. It should be used with care in patients with congestive heart failure, although reducing the heart rate may improve ventricular function (see earlier section on CHF, p. 90). The systemic clearance of propranolol is increased in hyperthyroid states and because of the continued presence of circulating thyroid hormone, propranolol must be continued for a week post thyroidectomy. Propranolol may be used in conjunction with iodides to prepare the mildly thyrotoxic patient for surgery. This approach is quicker (1–2 weeks), but abnormalities of the myocardium may not be corrected. Therefore it is still preferable to render the patient euthyroid with carbimazole.

If emergency surgery is required in a hyperthyroid patient, an intravenous infusion of esmolol (50–500 µg/kg), titrated to restore a normal heart rate, is recommended. Intravascular fluid volume and electrolyte balance should be restored. When diarrhoea is severe, dehydration must be corrected preoperatively. Atrial fibrillation and heart failure should be treated appropriately (see p. 97, 100).

Hypothyroidism

Hypothyroidism is frequently subclinical and, when this is the case, is associated with normal serum concentrations of thyroid hormones and mildly elevated serum TSH levels. In such cases, it may have little or no perioperative significance. In overt hypothyroidism the relative lack of thyroid hormones results in slow mental functions, dry skin, intolerance to cold, depression of ventilatory response to hypoxia and hypercarbia, impaired clearance of free water, slow gastric emptying, and bradycardia. In severe cases, cardiomegaly, heart failure, pericardial and pleural effusions are seen.

Ideal preoperative management of hypothyroidism consists of restoring a normal thyroid status, as these patients are extremely sensitive to anaesthetic agents and opiates. Severe hypotension and even cardiac arrest can occur with induction of anaesthesia. Adequate treatment of hypothyroidism (100–200 μg of *l*-thyroxine daily) takes time to achieve. The dose should be reduced to 25 μg daily in the elderly and those with cardiac disease. *l*-thyroxine should be continued on the day of surgery.

Myxoedema coma can be precipitated by stress in a hypothyroid patient and is associated with a high mortality. Management involves slow intravenous administration of *l*-thyroxine (50 μg) with continuous ECG monitoring followed by a further 25 μg eight-hourly. Other therapy includes maintenance of normothermia, intravenous fluids, hydrocortisone, and antibiotics. Addison's disease is more common in hypothyroid patients and some endocrinologists routinely treat non-iatrogenic hypothyroid patients with stress doses of steroid perioperatively. Hypothyroid patients with symptomatic CAD pose special problems. The need for thyroid therapy must be balanced against the risk of aggravating symptoms of ischaemia. In such patients, early coronary revascularisation should be considered.

Adrenal disease

Adrenocortical dysfunction

The adrenal cortex produces steroid hormones of which the glucocorticoids (such as cortisol) and mineralocorticoids (for example, aldosterone) are the most important. The secretion of most of the steroids is controlled by pituitary hormones, with adrenocorticotrophic hormone (ACTH) the most important.

Glucocorticoid excess (Cushing's syndrome) results from either endogenous oversecretion or chronic treatment with high-dose glucocorticoids. Preoperative considerations in such patients include regulating hyperglycaemia and hypertension and ensuring that the intravascular fluid volume and electrolyte concentrations are normal. Patients with Cushing's syndrome caused by an ACTH-secreting pituitary adenoma have an increased bleeding tendency and a raised central venous pressure, which should be monitored perioperatively.[31]

Patients on steroid medication will require perioperative supplementation if the total daily dose is equivalent to 10 mg/day prednisolone or more. All patients should take their normal oral dose of steroid medication on the day of surgery, with those undergoing intermediate and major surgery also needing an intravenous bolus of hydrocortisone (25 mg) on induction of anaesthesia. Further postoperative supplementation will be required in such patients in line with current recommendations.[28] Those patients treated with immunosuppressive doses must be maintained on their high dose perioperatively. Finally, patients taking less than 10 mg/day do not require additional steroid cover. See also Chapter 9.

Patients who have stopped steroid treatment in the last three months should be managed as described for those on current medication, whilst those who have stopped steroid treatment for more than three months do not require any supplementation.

Patients with Cushing's disease resulting from endogenous production of glucocorticoids do not require supplemental doses of steroids preoperatively, but it will be required postoperatively.[32]

Glucocorticoid deficiency can result from decreased secretion of ACTH, destruction of the adrenal cortex (for example, by haemorrhage, cancer or tuberculosis) or withdrawal of steroid therapy. Preoperative preparation of such patients includes treatment of hypovolaemia, hyperkalaemia, and hyponatraemia if present. Since these patients cannot respond to stressful situations, it seems appropriate that they should be given hydrocortisone supplementation (25 mg) intravenously every eight hours during the preioperative period, rather than the higher doses previously recommended.[33]

Primary hyperaldosteronism (Conn's syndrome) is a rare condition that leads to potassium depletion, sodium retention, muscle weakness, hypertension, tetany, polyuria, and inability to concentrate urine. Preoperatively, intravascular fluid volume, electrolyte concentrations, and renal function should be restored to within normal limits. Preoperative treatment with spironolactone (for at least two weeks) reduces hypertension and improves electrolyte status.

Phaeochromocytoma

Phaeochromocytoma is a catecholamine-producing tumour derived from chromaffin, which normally arises in the adrenal medulla but can occur anywhere in the body. Paroxysmal tachycardia, hypertension, sweating, and headaches are the cardinal symptoms. The reduction of mortality associated with surgical resection of a phaeochromocytoma is attributed to the use of α-adrenergic receptor blockade preoperatively.[34] α-adrenergic receptor blockade with prazosin or phenoxybenzamine (initially 10–20 mg twice daily) restores plasma volume by counteracting the vasoconstrictive effects of high levels of catecholamines; 10–14 days are required for the reexpansion of the blood volume to occur, along with control and stabilisation of the blood pressure. If tachycardia develops, a β-blocker (such as propranolol 40–80 mg daily) should be added. It is mandatory to institute α-adrenergic receptor blockade prior to administering β-blockers, otherwise unopposed α activity may occur, resulting in severe hypertension and arrhythmias. In patients with coronary heart disease, α-adrenergic blocking agents should be introduced cautiously to prevent sudden hypotension and tachycardia.

Occasionally, intravenous administration of α-adrenergic blockers may be required but this requires a minimum of three days treatment. Phenoxybenzamine is the treatment of choice, with an initial bolus dose (1 mg/kg) given intravenously followed by 1.5–2 mg/kg daily over the next two days. Propranolol (orally) should be added if the pulse rate increases above 120/min. Phenoxybenzamine (50 mg) and propranolol are given on the day of surgery. The effects of excess catecholamine secretion may be observed in other organ systems. Myocardial ischaemia, ventricular arrhythmias, and glucose intolerance should be appropriately treated. Preoperatively, direct arterial and central venous pressure monitoring should be instituted along with the other routine monitors.

Electrolyte disturbances

Electrolyte disturbances reflect the balance between body water and electrolytes. The minimum daily replacement values in the normal adult (70 kg) are 80 mmol sodium (Na^+), 80 mmol potassium (K^+), and 2.5–3.0 litres water. The osmolality of the extracellular and intracellular fluid are almost equal and can be estimated as:

$$2[Na^+] + [glucose] + [blood\ urea\ and\ nitrogen]$$

where the concentrations are expressed in mmol/l. The normal range of osmolality is 285–290 mOsm/kg. The osmotic threshold for thirst (300 mOsm/kg) is higher than for secretion of antidiuretic hormone (ADH). Therefore, thirst is an important sign of fluid depletion.

Hyponatraemia

Hyponatraemia can occur in three forms: isotonic (protein accumulation such as myeloma), hypertonic (hyperglycaemia; absorption of glycine during resection of prostate), and hypotonic. Hypotonic hyponatraemia can be divided further into hypovolaemic hyponatraemia (gastrointestinal losses), hypervolaemic hyponatraemia (cardiac failure, cirrhosis, nephrotic syndrome) and isovolaemic hyponatraemia (syndrome of inappropriate secretion of ADH). Hyponatraemia (serum levels less than 123 mmol/l) can cause cerebral oedema, coma, and convulsions.[35] Depending on the cause, treatment ranges from administration of hypertonic saline to restriction of fluids. The rate of rise of serum sodium should not exceed 1 mmol/l/h, as it may result in demyelination.[35] Cerebral oedema disappears at a serum sodium of 130 mmol/l and this is probably the acceptable lower limit for elective surgery.[31]

Hypernatraemia

Hypernatraemia is often iatrogenic (for example, failure to provide sufficient water to an unconscious patient). Neurological insults such as head injury and brain tumour can cause diabetes insipidus (DI); the lack of ADH results in raised serum osmolality and sodium levels. The management of DI includes desmopressin and fluid replacement (hypotonic fluids if the serum osmolality is greater than 290 mOsm/kg). Rapid correction of hypernatraemia can lead to cerebral oedema and convulsions, hence it should be undertaken slowly. Preoperatively, a serum sodium level of less than 150 mmol/l is acceptable.

Hypokalaemia

Inadequate intake of potassium, loop diuretic therapy, excessive gastrointestinal and renal losses, and shifts from extracellular to intracellular spaces are common causes of hypokalaemia. The preoperative management includes treatment of the cause as well as the deficiency. Either oral or intravenous potassium supplementation can be administered, depending upon the urgency. If the intravenous route is deemed necessary, it should be undertaken using continuous ECG monitoring. A preoperative serum potassium level above 2.9 mmol/l is acceptable provided treatment is ongoing.[31]

Hyperkalaemia

Hyperkalaemia results from various causes including renal failure, red blood cell haemolysis, muscle damage, and excess intake. The principal anaesthetic risk in such patients is abnormalities of cardiac function including electrical disturbances and poor contractility. Methods of reducing high serum potassium levels include intravenous administration of saline, glucose with insulin (1 unit per 2 g of glucose), kayexalate enemas (which binds potassium in the gut), and dialysis (in renal failure). An acceptable upper limit of serum potassium is 5.9 mmol/l.

Hypercalcaemia

The serum concentration of calcium and phosphorus are regulated by parathyroid hormone, calcitonin, and vitamin D. The normal total serum calcium level is 2.15–2.60 mmol/l, although the value is dependent upon the albumin level declining 0.02 mmol/l for each 1 g/l drop in albumin. The physiologically relevant measurement is that of ionised calcium, but this is less often performed.

Patients with moderate hypercalcaemia who have normal renal and cardiovascular function present no special preoperative problems. On occasions, a hypercalcaemic patient may be severely dehydrated and the raised calcium levels can precipitate serious arrhythmias. The ECG should be examined for evidence of a shortened QT interval with an absent ST, as this is associated with hypercalcaemia.

Management of hypercalcaemia includes correcting the dehydration, enhancing renal excretion of calcium, and inhibiting bone resorption. Once the underlying fluid deficit has been corrected with intravenous isotonic saline (3–4 l/day), frusemide should be given to help reduce the serum calcium level further as it increases renal calcium excretion. Thiazide diuretics should not be used as they cause increased tubular reabsorption of calcium. Increased diuresis can cause hypomagnesaemia and hypokalaemia and these need correcting as appropriate. Hypophosphataemia decreases the uptake of calcium by bone, thus stimulating bone breakdown leading to further increases in serum calcium. Therefore, phosphate should be given to restore normal serum phosphate levels. Hydration and diuresis, accompanied by phosphate repletion, suffice in the management of most patients with hypercalcaemia. If additional interventions are needed to correct hypercalcaemia, glucocorticoids, mithramycin, and calcitonin may be given.[31] Finally, specific therapy for inhibiting osteoclast-mediated bone resorption includes the use of biphosphonates, plicamycin, and calcitonin.[30]

Hypocalcaemia
Hypoparathyroidism and chronic renal failure are the main causes of hypocalcaemia. Hypocalcaemia can give rise to cardiac arrhythmias, decreased myocardial contractility, tetany (especially with hyperventilation), laryngeal stridor, and convulsions. A prolonged QT interval may be found on the ECG. Patients with symptomatic hypocalcaemia should be treated with intravenous calcium gluconate (10%, 10–20 ml) by slow infusion followed by an infusion (0.5–2 mg calcium/kg/h) with monitoring of calcium levels. The serum levels of magnesium[36] and phosphate should also be measured in these patients and hypomagnesaemia, which usually co-exists, can be corrected acutely by the intravenous administration of magnesium (1–2 g).

Gastrointestinal and liver disease

Although preoperative preparation of the gastrointestinal (GI) tract is usually the responsibility of the surgeon, GI diseases can cause derangements in other systems which can affect the safety of anaesthesia. Patients with disorders of the GI system may have marked alterations in fluids, electrolytes, and nutrition and these should be optimised preoperatively. Liver disease is often associated with GI disease and can, in itself, lead to severe haemostatic derangements which should be corrected preoperatively.

Intestinal obstruction

Up to 8 litres of fluid is secreted by the GI tract every 24 hours, most of which is reabsorbed. Thus, severe dehydration follows loss of GI fluids as a consequence of vomiting and sequestration into oedematous tissues and the abdominal cavity secondary to ischaemia of the bowel wall. In addition, severe electrolyte imbalances occur, although the exact nature of these depends upon the site of the obstruction.

Fluid losses

The loss of fluid leads to a reduction in the extracellular fluid (ECF) compartment; external losses, which can include that from vomiting, are responsible for the most serious losses, although internal losses may account for 10–15% of body weight (7–10 l). Assessment of the adequacy of intravascular volume begins at the bedside. A patient with a moderate deficit of ECF volume (6–8% of body weight or 4–6 l) is apathetic, with dry mucous membranes, poor skin turgor, tachycardia, and orthostatic hypotension. A patient with a severe deficit resulting from the loss of 10% of body weight (7–8 l) will be stuporous, tachycardic, and hypotensive when supine. Routine laboratory investigations do not enable volume losses to be accurately measured although the haemoglobin concentration and haematocrit rise with severe ECF volume loss and the urea may rise secondary to reduced renal blood flow.

Electrolyte losses

Obstruction of the upper GI tract at or near the pylorus produces repetitive vomiting with loss of hydrogen ions (H^+), chloride ions (Cl^-), and water. The alkaline secretions of the pancreas and duodenum are retained and therefore the loss of H^+ leads to a metabolic alkalosis. Potassium (K^+) is also lost as a result of renal compensatory mechanisms. Small bowel obstruction presents a different picture as the alkaline pancreatic and duodenal fluids are also lost. Large volumes of both electrolytes and fluids may be lost in such patients; indeed, they may present with circulatory collapse.

Preoperative optimisation of these patients includes the insertion of a wide-bore nasogastric tube to empty the stomach and this helps prevent further vomiting. It also decompresses the bowel, so reducing the incidence of ischaemic necrosis. The fluid loss should be estimated on clinical grounds, as outlined above, and should be replaced using 0.9% saline which replaces Na^+, Cl^-, and water. K^+ should also be added if hypokalaemia is present (see above). As indicated earlier, the fluid loss may be significant and therefore large volumes of intravenous fluids may be required; rapid replacement (2–3 l/h) is well tolerated unless the patient has underlying cardiac or renal disease. The adequacy of the volume replacement will include the regular assessment of pulse rate, blood pressure, and urine output. In the severely dehydrated patient or in patients with cardiac disease, a central venous catheter may provide further information on the adequacy of the fluid resuscitation. Attempts at insertion should not be made until reasonable fluid resuscitation has occurred, because of the technical difficulty associated with their insertion in the dehydrated patient and the consequent increased risk of collateral damage to important structures.

Adequate fluid resuscitation is essential before the induction of anaesthesia and, ideally, a urine output of 0.5–1 ml/kg/h should be achieved before surgery is considered appropriate. Pain frequently accompanies intestinal obstruction and this may influence the pulse rate and blood pressure values.

Hiatus hernia

Patients with a known hiatus hernia are at increased risk of regurgitating on induction of anaesthesia and consequently are at greater risk of pulmonary aspiration. A number of different preoperative treatment regimes have been proposed for these patients and it is generally believed that a reduced gastric volume and/or increased gastric pH are the ways in which the risk of pulmonary aspiration can be reduced. There are, however, no data to show improvements after the use of antacid therapy, H_2-receptor antagonists, proton pump inhibitors or prokinetics. Further, prophylactic measures can cause unwanted side effects. Thus, little can be done preoperatively, aside from ensuring that the gastric volume is minimised non-pharmacologically and that care is taken to minimise the risk of airway soiling during anaesthesia.[37]

Liver disease

The recognition of occult or overt liver disease, as well as efforts to normalise the hepatic function, is essential to reduce associated perioperative morbidity and mortality. It is important to recognise that patients with severe hepatic disease are extreme risks for surgery, often more so than those with cardiac disease. There are numerous causes of acute and chronic liver disease but the most common in Western society is cirrhosis. The Child–Pugh[38] classification grades liver disease according to increasing severity (from A to C) on the basis of certain parameters (Table 6.2). Preoperative management of patients with hepatic disease requires an understanding of the modifiable risk factors which can be optimised before surgery.[39,40]

Coagulopathy
All procoagulation factors are derived from the liver, with the exception of von Willebrand factor. Since the half-lives of some of these factors are short, disorders of coagulation set in rapidly in patients with hepatic dysfunction. Impaired bile secretion (resulting from, for example, fulminant liver failure or obstructive jaundice) leads to a deficiency of vitamin K-dependent factors (II, VII, IX, and X). The liver is also responsible for the clearance of activated coagulation products and failure to remove these complexes leads

117

Table 6.2 The Child–Pugh classification of liver disease (reproduced with permission from reference[38])

	A	B	C
Bilirubin (mmol/l)	<40	40–50	>50
Albumin (g/l)	>35	28–35	<28
Ascites	None	Mild	Moderate-severe
Encephalopathy	Absent	Grade I, II	Grade III,IV
PT prolonged (sec)	0	<2.5	>2.5
Surgical risk	Good	Moderate	Poor
Postoperative mortality (%)	3–10	10–30	50–80

PT, prothrombin time

to factor consumption. Further, the liver is the site of production of important anticoagulant and fibrinolytic factors and finally, platelet quality and quantity may suffer in hepatic disease. Hence, the coagulopathy in hepatic dysfunction is multifactorial.

Parenteral vitamin K (10 mg/day) can be administered if the prothrombin time (PT) is prolonged. Correction of an abnormal PT by vitamin K only occurs in patients with severe malabsorption, those on neomycin bowel regimens or those with obstructive liver disease. If the surgery is urgent or if the PT does not return to normal after vitamin K, fresh frozen plasma (FFP) (5–8 ml/kg) can be used during surgery. Decreased levels of coagulation factors do not require replacement unless the patient is actively bleeding (before or during the surgery).

Cardiovascular disturbances
A variety of cardiovascular effects are produced by liver disease. Portovenous and arteriovenous shunting of blood is associated with severe liver disease (for reasons that are not known)[41] and these lead to an increased resting cardiac output. A low systemic vascular resistance also occurs. Coupled with these changes is an increase in plasma volume. Fortunately, patients with cirrhosis have a reduced incidence of arteriosclerosis, unless the patient is also a heavy smoker.

Hypovolaemia and anaemia must be corrected as decreased oxygen delivery to a hyperdynamic myocardium may lead to myocardial ischaemia. Congestive heart failure is also associated with liver disease and should be treated if present. There is increased risk of bacterial endocarditis in patients with portosystemic shunting and such patients need antibiotic prophylaxis prior to surgery.

Oesophageal varices are frequently present in such patients. It has been shown that there is a low risk of variceal bleeding from oesophageal instrumentation (for example, nasogastric tube insertion, endoscopy). In the event of acute variceal bleeding, the preoperative insertion of a Sengstaken-Blakemore tube may be a life-saving manoeuvre.

Pulmonary disturbances

Intrapulmonary shunting may be present in patients with severe cirrhosis, leading to low PaO_2 values. Pleural effusions may also occur and, in association with ascites, will cause further hypoxia as a result of mechanical constriction of pulmonary function. Pleural effusions should be tapped preoperatively and ascites treated appropriately (see later). Patients with liver disease frequently smoke and this further compounds problems with gas exchange. Physiotherapy and other treatments for chronic lung disease may be needed.

Renal disturbances

Renal insufficiency may occur with acute, chronic or obstructive hepatic diseases. In obstructive jaundice, biliary products excreted through the kidney can lead to acute tubular necrosis (ATN) as bile salts are toxic to tubular epithelium. The incidence of renal failure as a result of ATN is reduced by maintaining a urine flow of 1 ml/kg/h, using isotonic saline and mannitol before and during the surgery.[42] A common cause of acute renal insufficiency in hospitalised patients with hepatic failure is aggressive diuresis, which presents with increased creatinine and decreased urine volume and sodium. Judicious use of salt-free albumin, or 0.45% sodium chloride, will improve the urine output.

The true "hepatorenal syndrome" is a progressive oliguric renal failure seen in patients with cirrhosis, hepatoma or acute hepatitis. It appears to be a functional lesion as pathological examination does not reveal any consistent changes. It often follows a sudden loss of effective blood volume after GI bleeding, paracentesis or vigorous diuresis. Preoperative hepatorenal syndrome has been associated with nearly 100% mortality, in operations other than liver transplantation. Haemodialysis and arteriovenous haemofiltration have been used to temporarily manage hepatorenal syndrome during fulminant, but reversible, hepatic disease or until liver transplantation can be achieved.[43]

Ascites

Ascites is one of the more common manifestations of liver failure and its presence indicates severe liver disease. The presence of ascites in a patient indicates that they are at greater risk of surgery than those without.[41] Treatment of patients with ascites awaiting surgery includes sodium restriction (less than 1 g per day), discontinuation of prostaglandin inhibitors such as aspirin and indomethacin, and administration of the potassium-sparing diuretic spironolactone.[44] If spironolactone does not induce diuresis, frusemide may be used with care – too rapid diuresis is an important cause of hepatic failure in such patients and, ideally, these measures should be commenced early. Little can be done for the patient requiring emergency surgery.

Electrolyte disturbances

Hyponatraemia and hypokalaemia are common in patients with cirrhosis when ascites is present. Administration of normal saline may correct hyponatraemia, but may increase the ascites. Administration of salt-poor albumin and frusemide can enhance free water clearance. Hypokalaemia should be avoided in these patients and is corrected by administering enteral (or parenteral) potassium.

Encephalopathy

Hepatic encephalopathy is an indicator of increased postoperative mortality. It results from raised levels of plasma ammonia, which is absorbed from the GI tract but is not converted to urea by the diseased liver. Management is focused on decreasing the urea-splitting organisms in the gut, reducing the protein load in the gut lumen and suppressing transport mechanisms for ammonia across the gut wall.[40] Lactulose is an unabsorbable disaccharide that acidifies intraluminal pH and traps ammonium ion (NH_4+) in the colon. Neomycin inhibits replication of the ammoniogenic colonic flora, but may be nephrotoxic in these patients. The protein load is reduced by suction removal of intragastric blood, a low protein diet and catharsis to purge bacteria and blood products from the gut.

Nutritional support

If surgery is not urgent, nutritional supplementation is a major part of the preoperative preparation and this requires the involvement of a dietician.

Haematological disease

Anaemia

Anaemia, or a decreased level of haemoglobin, leads to a reduction in arterial oxygen-carrying capacity. In acute anaemia, reductions in arterial oxygen content lead to compensatory increases in cardiac output, while in chronic anaemia, oxygen delivery is facilitated through increased 2,3-diphosphoglycerate levels in the red blood cells. Clinically acceptable oxygen transport can be sustained at haemoglobin levels of 7–8 g/dl[45,46] provided the patient has a normal intravascular volume and normal cardiovascular responses.

The preoperative preparation of an anaemic patient depends upon the cause of the anaemia and the urgency of surgery. In an otherwise fit, mildly anaemic patient requiring elective surgery, it is preferable to search for the underlying cause of the anaemia first (to exclude malignancy) before surgery is performed. In iron deficiency anaemia, optimal oral ferrous sulphate supplements may raise the haemoglobin by 1 g per week and iron preload for four weeks prior to surgery may be beneficial in reducing the fall in haemoglobin concentration postoperatively.[47] This is obviously not possible if the surgery is urgent, when a decision has to be made as to whether preoperative transfusion is indicated. Historically, a haematocrit less than 30% (or haemoglobin less than 10 g/dl) was the trigger for preoperative blood transfusion.[48] A lower baseline haemoglobin level is now considered acceptable, principally because of the recognised hazards of blood transfusion. Red blood cell transfusion should not be dictated by a single haemoglobin value, but should be based on the patient's risks of developing complications of inadequate oxygenation.[48] Red blood cell transfusion is rarely indicated when the haemoglobin concentration is greater than 10 g/dl and is almost always indicated when it is less than 6 g /dl.[48]

The decision to transfuse a specific patient should take into consideration the duration of anaemia, the intravascular volume, the extent of the operation, the probability of massive blood loss, and the presence of existing conditions such as impaired pulmonary function and myocardial ischaemia.

If preoperative transfusion is required, it is preferable to complete the transfusion 24 hours before surgery, to allow time for depleted 2,3-diphosphoglycerate in stored red cells to be restored. Smoking should be prohibited, to reduce the amount of carboxyhaemoglobin which reduces oxygen carriage. In emergency surgery, blood replacement therapy may be required immediately preoperatively to help maintain both intravascular volume and minimally acceptable haemoglobin levels.

Haemoglobinopathies

Haemoglobinopathies are caused by genetically determined abnormalities of the globin chain and they can be classified into two broad groups. In one group there is the production of an abnormal chain, for example, sickle cell disease, whilst in the other group there is abnormal production of a normal chain, for example, thalassaemia.

Sickle cell disease

Sickle cell disease is a complex clinical entity, inherited as an autosomal recessive trait where there is a single amino acid substitution (glutamine to valine) on position 6 of the β chain. This causes polymerisation of the reduced haemoglobin, leading to "sickling" of the red blood cells, resulting in vasoocclusion; this is the single most important pathophysiological process and causes most of the acute complications.[49] This tendency is increased by a rise in temperature, acidosis, dehydration, and hypoxia and is more common in homozygous individuals (SS genotype).

The incidence of sickle cell disease is high amongst patients of Afro-Caribbean descent and all suspected patients must be screened preoperatively. Although the "Sickledex" test is simple to perform it is not

121

specific and therefore haemoglobin electrophoresis is the test of choice to identify the genotype.[50] Surgery is a time of particular risk for patients with sickle cell disease and it has been standard practice to consider preoperative transfusion but this adds transfusion-related risks. Current recommendations are that a relatively conservative transfusion programme should be followed in patients undergoing intermediate or high-risk elective procedures, aiming to raise the haemoglobin to above 10 g/dl, whilst for minor procedures there appears to be little benefit from transfusion. In contrast, patients requiring emergency surgery are at the greatest risk of perioperative complications and optimal transfusion support needs to be discussed with the haematologist.[49] It is essential that intravenous fluids are administered to these patients during preoperative starvation so as to avoid hypovolaemia, dehydration, and hyperosmolality. Heavy premedication, causing cardiorespiratory depression, is also best avoided.

Abnormalities of haemostasis in surgical patients

Haemostatic abnormalities commonly encountered in the perioperative period may be acquired or inherited. Acquired coagulation disorders may be secondary to liver disease, vitamin K deficiency, the use of anticoagulant drugs or following massive blood transfusion. Commonly encountered inherited disorders of clotting include haemophilia A (a defect in factor VIII activity) and von Willebrand's disease (a defect in von Willebrand's component of factor VIII).

The tests of coagulation include the prothrombin time (PT), the activated partial thromboplastin time (PTT), and the thrombin time (TT). The PT reflects the activity of factors I, II, V, VII, and X and is prolonged when there is less than 30% activity of these factors and in vitamin K deficiency and liver disease (see earlier section on liver disease, p. 107, for more details on related coagulopathy). The PTT reflects the activity of factors I, II, V, VIII, IX, X, XI, and XII and it is prolonged by heparin. The TT measures conversion of fibrinogen to fibrin and is prolonged by low fibrinogen levels, dysfibrinogenaemia, the use of heparin and by fibrin degradation products (FDPs) interfering with fibrin polymerisation.

It is prudent to seek the advice of the haematologist when optimising patients with coagulation abnormalities preoperatively.

Acquired coagulation disorders
Coagulopathy and massive transfusion. This is unusual before 1–1.5 times the blood volume has been replaced and reasons include thrombocytopenia and a deficiency of clotting factors. Clinical bleeding is unlikely if the platelet count is above 50 000 cells/mm³. However, following the loss of one blood volume, platelets should be available and transfused if there is evidence of prolonged bleeding. In adults, 5–10 units of platelets per blood

volume are required, whilst in children the value is 0.3 unit/kg. Bleeding from factor deficiency after massive transfusion is usually due to diminished levels of fibrinogen (less than 75 mg/dl) and labile factors (V, VIII, IX). Cryoprecipitate contains primarily fibrinogen, factor VIII, and von Willebrand's factor and is indicated when fibrinogen levels are less than 100 mg/dl (10 units of cryoprecipitate increase fibrinogen levels by about 100 mg/dl). Labile clotting factors are administered as fresh frozen plasma.

Disseminated intravascular coagulation (DIC). DIC can be caused by various insults and is characterised by both the diffuse formation of fibrin clots and enhanced fibrinolysis. The resultant picture is one of bleeding due to consumption of the clotting factors, thrombocytopenia, and increased fibrin degradation products. Treatment of DIC involves controlling the precipitating cause in association with transfusion of appropriate blood products (for example FFP, platelets, and cryoprecipitate).

Management of patients taking anticoagulant drugs. Such drugs include heparin (venous thromboembolism prophylaxis), oral warfarin (prosthetic heart valves and atrial fibrillation), and low-dose aspirin (antiplatelet action).

- The anticoagulation effect of heparin is normally reversed 2–4 hours after the drug is stopped. If faster reversal is required, protamine (1 mg for every 100 units of heparin remaining in the patient) can be used intravenously.[51]
- Warfarin is a vitamin K antagonist with a long half-life (35 hours) and needs to be discontinued 2–4 days preoperatively. Reversal of anticoagulation can be accomplished more rapidly with the administration of vitamin K (effective in 3–6 hours) or FFP (5–15 ml/kg). The current practice of interrupting oral warfarin in patients with prosthetic heart valves preoperatively and covering the perioperative period with heparin has been challenged.[52] Interruption of warfarin can give rise to periods of rebound hypercoagulability, caused by a delayed rise in protein C and S. Heparin may compound this by causing aggregation of platelets, resulting in an increased risk of valve thrombosis. However, the practice of discontinuation of warfarin preoperatively and institution of heparin if the risk of thrombotic complication is high is widely used.[53] Further prospective trials are clearly required to define the risks and benefits of this practice. Patients having minor cutaneous surgery can be managed without interruption of warfarin. There are reports of transurethral resection of the prostate using laser ablation technique being carried out successfully in patients on warfarin therapy.
- All non-steroidal antiinflammatory drugs (NSAIDs), with the exception of aspirin, reversibly inhibit platelet aggregation by interfering with the cyclooxygenase pathway. The duration of inhibition is dependent upon the

half-life of the individual NSAID.[51,54] Aspirin is thought to permanently inhibit this pathway and as the half-life of platelets in circulation is approximately four days, 7–10 days are required before platelet function returns to normal. There are reports that suggest this length of time is excessive and that the antiplatelet action of aspirin is reversed in 48 hours.[55]

Other drugs affecting coagulation. These include tissue plasminogen activator (tPA) and streptokinase.

- tPA is a naturally occurring enzyme that converts plasminogen into its active form, plasmin, which lyses fibrin clots. It is used to treat acute occlusion of coronary, cerebral, pulmonary, and peripheral arteries and has a very short half-life (a few minutes only). However, fibrinogen levels remain depressed for up to 36 hours after stopping the drug. If emergency surgery is required after tPA therapy, it should be delayed for a minimum of 20–30 minutes and FFP or cryoprecipitate given to correct the hypofibrinogenaemia.
- Streptokinase is an indirect activator of plasminogen and the ongoing fibrinolysis stops within a few hours of stopping the streptokinase infusion. Fibrinogen levels may remain low for up to 36 hours.

Congenital coagulation disorders

Congenital disorders of coagulation, such as haemophilia A and von Willebrand's disease, are occasionally encountered in anaesthetic practice.

Haemophilia A. The severity of bleeding complications depends upon the degree of deficiency of factor VIII coagulation activity. Management of these patients requiring surgery includes assay of factor level, knowledge of preparations of coagulation components available and the requirements for the surgical procedure. The normal level of coagulation activity of factor VIII is defined as 1 IU/ml and the actual level is expressed as a percent of normal activity. Activity levels greater than 40% are recommended before surgery is commenced.[56] A dose of 1 IU/kg of factor VIII raises the activity by 2%. The half-life of factor VIII is 6–10 hours and factor levels must be checked before and after administration of factors; 10% of haemophiliacs develop antibodies that inactivate factor VIII. Patients with resistance must be treated with high-dose factor VIII, activated factor IX or by plasmapheresis.[57]

Von Willebrand's disease. Von Willebrand's factor (vWF) serves as an anchor for platelet adhesion to collagen and protects and stabilises factor VIII. Deficiency of vWF leads to prolonged bleeding time. Infusion of cryoprecipitate or factor VIII concentrate is needed to normalise platelet function. Desmopressin (0.3 μg/kg) increases endothelial cell release of von

Willebrand's factor, factor VIII, and plasminogen activator and its use may be beneficial.[58]

Renal disease

Patients with renal disease fall into one of two categories: patients with end-stage disease on dialysis and patients with renal dysfunction not requiring dialysis.

Dialysis patients with end-stage renal disease

The physiological abnormalities encountered in patients with end-stage renal disease are anaemia, bleeding abnormalities, cardiovascular dysfunction, altered blood volume status, electrolyte and metabolic disturbances, susceptibility to infections, and altered response to drugs.

Anaemia

Serum haematocrit values of less than 30% are commonly encountered in these patients as a result of inadequate production of erythropoietin. Routine erythrocyte transfusions are not indicated if the anaemia is chronic and well tolerated. Acutely decreased preoperative haematocrit values require investigation for other causes of anaemia, in all patients except those requiring life-saving surgery. Exogenous administration of human recombinant erythropoietin can correct the anaemia of chronic renal failure,[59] but its use is not widespread.

Coagulation abnormalities

Uraemic patients are at risk of increased bleeding. If measured, bleeding time may be prolonged and the platelet count will be mildly decreased. PT and PTT are normal in patients with uraemia and any deviation from normal should be investigated preoperatively. One of the reasons for the increased bleeding tendency in these patients is the abnormal platelet function and it has been shown that dialysis reduces this platelet dysfunction. It is advisable, therefore, to dialyse such patients within 24 hours of surgery.[60]

Other haemostatic options in patients with uraemia include use of desmopressin, cryoprecipitate, and conjugated oestrogen. These agents, through unknown mechanisms, shorten the bleeding time. Desmopressin is safe and well tolerated in uraemic patients and has a more rapid onset of action than oestrogen therapy. Unlike cryoprecipitate, it is not associated with infectious complications.[61]

Patients requiring dialysis have an increased incidence of mucosal inflammatory changes in the gastrointestinal tract.[62] Histamine H_2-receptor antagonist drugs, antacids or sucralfate may be indicated during the perioperative period, as these patients may be at increased risk of GI bleeding.

Cardiovascular and blood volume abnormalities

Cardiovascular management and intravascular fluid balance are difficult in patients on dialysis because of preexisting myocardial dysfunction, the presence of coronary artery disease, arteriovenous shunts, and autonomic dysfunction. As with any patient undergoing surgery, maintenance of intravascular volume is mandatory. Patients undergoing preoperative ultra-filtration are particularly at risk as this increases the risk of hypovolaemia. Invasive haemodynamic monitoring may be needed to guide volume replacement. Normal saline solution free of potassium supplements should be used.

The location and patency of the arteriovenous fistula or shunt used for dialysis should be noted and the use of that extremity should be avoided for blood pressure monitoring and placement of intravascular catheters.

Electrolyte abnormalities

Patients should be dialysed within 24 hours of elective surgery to eliminate toxic waste products, control metabolic acidosis and maintain body water and serum electrolyte levels. The serum potassium should be measured immediately preoperatively and compared with the usual predialysis value to determine the level of hyperkalaemia that is normally tolerated by the patient. If it is high, further dialysis, or other forms of therapy to treat hyper-kalaemia, may be required (see earlier, p. 114). Patients with a serum bicarbonate below 12–15 mmol/l should be investigated for ketoacidosis or lactic acidosis. A mildly elevated magnesium, which may be present even after effective dialysis, does not appear to be clinically significant.

Susceptibility to infections

Infectious complications are a leading cause of perioperative mortality in dialysis-dependent patients, hence aseptic techniques are mandatory during intravascular cannulations. As the incidence of hepatitis B and C is high among these patients, effective measures must be taken to ensure the operator is protected from contamination by blood and secretions.

Pharmacological alterations

The loss of renal mechanisms for drug elimination, biochemical abnormal-ities resulting from uraemia that alter drug bioavailability and the effects of dialysis on drug elimination all contribute to altered pharmacokinetics. Potential pharmacokinetic changes should be identified preoperatively.

Patients with renal dysfunction not requiring dialysis

The preoperative management of patients with renal dysfunction should be directed towards preserving the existing renal function and also to detecting and treating any acute deterioration in renal function. Serum levels of blood urea, nitrogen (BUN), and creatinine must be estimated and compared with previous values to detect any decrease in renal function. If acute deterioration is detected preoperatively, the cause and reversibility must be assessed before the surgery and corrective measures taken. Surgical procedures that compromise renal perfusion (aortic cross clamping, cardiopulmonary bypass), especially in those with diabetes and poor myocardial function, can worsen renal dysfunction. Use of "renal protective agents" such as dopamine, frusemide, and mannitol should be considered.[63]

Patients with chronic renal failure (CRF) are salt and fluid restricted and many clinicians believe that a "well-filled" intravascular space will minimise any perioperative decrease in GFR. It has been suggested that, in CRF patients with stable cardiac function, diuretics are stopped and salt intake liberalised.[64] Maintenance of an adequate intravascular volume is probably the most effective way of preserving renal perfusion and thus preventing further deterioration in renal function. Optimising preoperative intravenous therapy in these patients is therefore important.

Neurological disease

This heterogeneous group of disorders includes diseases of the peripheral and central nervous system. Most of these diseases are chronic and patients may have complications resulting from long-term generalised muscle weakness. Reduced respiratory function and difficulty with mobilisation are particularly important in the perioperative period.

Parkinson's disease

This is one of the most common neurological conditions seen in elderly patients. Ideopathic Parkinson's results from a deficiency of dopamine in the substantia nigra and, as a consequence, a relative excess of acetylcholine stimulation in the corpus striatum. Levodopa, the precursor for endogenous dopamine, is effective in alleviating the symptoms of tremor, rigidity, and akinesia. Many patients are also treated with carbidopa, a peripheral dopa-decarboxylase inhibitor, in an attempt to reduce the peripheral effects of dopamine synthesis, particularly cardiac rhythm disturbances (including sinus tachycardia, AF and ventricular ectopics). Levodopa and carbidopa should be continued before surgery to avoid the return of Parkinson's symptoms.[65] Provided the patient's symptoms are well controlled by these drugs, they should tolerate anaesthesia and surgery well.[66] The more severely affected patient may prove difficult to assess preoperatively and may be very difficult to mobilise postoperatively. This will increase the perioperative risks in such patients and it is important to consider whether the benefits of the proposed surgery outweigh the risks.

Myasthenia gravis

Myasthenia gravis (MG) is an autoimmune disease of the neuromuscular junction characterised by a depletion of postsynaptic acetylcholine receptors (AchR), giving rise to the characteristic muscle weakness that is exacerbated by exercise and improved by rest. The disease may be localised or generalised and mild or severe, with the most severely affected developing bulbar and respiratory muscle weakness.[67,68]

MG is often associated with morphological abnormalities of the thymus and adults with generalised MG should undergo thymectomy, which alone produces an improvement in 60–70% of patients. This is the treatment of choice in young adults. Other medical treatment is aimed at improving neuromuscular transmission by the use of anticholinesterases, suppression of the immune system by the use of high-dose steroids and immunosuppressants (such as azathioprine) and, on occasions, by the use of plasmapheresis to reduce circulating antibodies to AchR. Anticholinesterases (such as neostigmine and pyridostigmine) were the mainstay of treatment but they only provide symptomatic relief and their long-term administration is associated with undesirable changes in the configuration of the acetylcholine receptors at the neuromuscular junction. Immunosuppression, if used, needs to be continued indefinitely, a significant disadvantage especially in the young. Plasmapheresis reduces circulating AchR antibodies very effectively, producing remission within a few days by allowing effective regeneration of acetylcholine receptors. It is, however, costly.

Anaesthetic management of the myasthenic patient must be individualised, taking into account the severity of the disease and the type of surgery. Preoperative respiratory function tests should be performed on patients with severe disease, to help identify those who may benefit from elective postoperative ventilation. Anticholinergic therapy potentiates vagal responses and hence adequate doses of atropine must be used to counter this effect. They also inhibit plasma cholinesterase activity and can decrease the metabolism of ester local anaesthetics and succinylcholine. Anticholinesterase therapy should be continued in those patients who are well controlled on small doses, whilst it is probably best discontinued in all other patients preoperatively. Older patients may benefit from the addition of corticosteroids and azathioprine preoperatively if their response to anticholinesterases is poor.[67] Those patients on high-dose steroid therapy should have this maintained preoperatively. Plasmapheresis may be used in those patients with severe disease who are not responding to other therapies.

Premedication with depressant drugs should be used with caution in those patients with MG who have little respiratory reserve and avoided completely in patients with bulbar symptoms.

Multiple sclerosis

Multiple sclerosis (MS) is characterised by acute episodes of neurological deficit appearing irregularly throughout the central nervous system (both in time and place) with spontaneous but partial remission. It results from demyelination of the white matter of the brain and spinal cord, especially the optic nerves, brainstem, cerebellar peduncles, and pyramidal tracts. Clinical features depend upon the extent of involvement. Sensory loss and ocular disturbances are the usual initial symptoms, but motor fibres (muscle weakness), respiratory centre dysfunction (abnormal respiratory drive) and autonomic dysfunction (hypotension) can also occur.

Patients with advanced MS may require frequent surgery for orthopaedic, urological, and neurological complications. Stress may exacerbate symptoms and adequate anxiolysis is required preoperatively. Hyperthermia should also be avoided preoperatively as this is known to exacerbate symptoms. Those with significant muscle atrophy are at risk of hyperkalaemia following the use of succinylcholine. Concern about possible neurotoxicity following the use of local anaesthetic agents in the spinal canal limits their use, although they have been used safely in parturients.[69]

Conclusion

The extent to which optimum preoperative preparation of the patient can occur depends upon the urgency of surgery, as well as the severity of the disease state. Every effort should be made to optimise treatment prior to surgery to help reduce perioperative morbidity. Our understanding of disease processes and their effect on other systems continues to expand and it is important that, where possible, we seek the advice of other medical colleagues to ensure that optimum care is provided to each and every patient in the perioperative period. As "perioperative physicians", anaesthetists are best placed to bring this knowledge together and apply it for the maximum benefit of individual patients.

1   Wilson J, Woods I, Fawcett J et al. Reducing the risk of major elective surgery: randomised controlled trial of preoperative optimisation of oxygen delivery. BMJ 1999; **318**: 1099–103.
2   Wallace A, Layug B, Tateo I et al. Prophylactic atenolol reduces postoperative myocardial ischaemia. Anesthesiology 1998; **88**: 7–17.
3   Berlauk JF, Abrams JH, Gilmour IJ et al. Preoperative optimisation of cardiovascular haemodynamics improves outcome in peripheral vascular surgery: a prospective, randomised clinical trial. Ann Surg 1991; **214**: 289–99.
4   Golman L, Caldera D, Nussbaum SR et al. Multifactorial index of cardiac risk in noncardiac surgical procedures. N Engl J Med 1977; **297**: 845–50.
5   Eagle KA, Brundage BH, Chaitman BR et al. Guidelines for perioperative cardiovascular evaluation for noncardiac surgery. Report of the American College of Cardiology/American Heart Association task force on practice guidelines. Circulation 1996; **93**: 1278–317.

6 Rao TLK, Jacobs KH, El-Etr AA. Reinfarction following anesthesia in patients with myocardial infarction. *Anesthesiology* 1983; **59**: 499–505.

7 Fleisher LA, Barash PG. Preoperative cardiac evaluation for noncardiac surgery: a functional approach. *Anesth Analg* 1992; **74**: 586–98.

8 Sonksen J, Gray R, Hutton P. Safer non-cardiac surgery for patients with coronary artery disease (editorial). *BMJ* 1999; **317**: 1400–1.

9 Cleland JGF, McGowan J, Clark A, Freemantle N. The evidence for β blockers in heart failure (editorial). *BMJ* 1999; **318**: 824–5.

10 Driscoll P, Gwinnutt C, Mackway-Jones K, Wardle T. *Advanced cardiac life support*, 2nd edn. London: Chapman and Hall Medical, 1997.

11 English KM, Channer KS. Managing atrial fibrillation in elderly people (editorial). *BMJ* 1999; **318**: 1088–9.

12 Prystowsky EN, Benson W, Fuster V *et al.* Management of patients with atrial fibrillation. A statement for healthcare professionals from the subcommittee on electrocardiography and electrophysiology, American Heart Association. *Circulation* 1996; **93**: 1262–77.

13 Goldman L, Caldera DL. Risks of general anaesthesia and elective operation in the hypertensive patient. *Anesthesiology* 1979; **50**: 285–92.

14 Prys-Roberts C, Meloche R, Foëx P. Studies of anaesthesia in relation to hypertension. I: Cardiovascular responses to treated and untreated patients. *Br J Anaesth* 1971; **43**: 122–37.

15 Ramsay LE, Williams B, Johnson GD *et al.* British Hypertension Society guidelines for hypertension management 1999: summary. *BMJ* 1999; **319**: 630–5.

16 Marcucci C, Fleisher LA. Hypertension: implications for anaesthetic management. *Curr Opin Anaesthesiol* 1997; **10**: 229–33.

17 Moudgil GC. The patient with reactive airways disease. *Can J Anaesth* 1997; **44**: 5/R77–R83.

18 Kingston HGG, Hirschman CA. Perioperative management of the patient with asthma. *Anesth Analg* 1984; **63**: 844–55.

19 Lipworth BJ. Modern drug treatment of chronic asthma. *BMJ* 1999; **318**: 380–4.

20 Lipworth BJ. Treatment of acute asthma. *Lancet* 1997; **350** (suppl II): 18–23.

21 Allen S. Management of the patient with asthma. *Curr Opin Anaesthesiol* 1996; **9**: 254–8.

22 Cohen MM, Cameron CB. Should you cancel the operation when a child has an upper respiratory tract infection? *Anesth Analg* 1991; **72**: 282–8.

23 Kerstjens HAM on behalf of *Clinical Evidence*. Stable chronic obstructive pulmonary disease. *BMJ* 1999; **319**: 495–500.

24 Nel MR, Morgan M. Smoking and anaesthesia (editorial). *Anaesthesia* 1996; **51**: 309–11.

25 Munday IT, Desai PM, Marshall CA *et al.* The effectiveness of pre-operative advice to stop smoking: a prospective controlled trial. *Anaesthesia* 1993; **48**: 816–18.

26 Stoelting RK. Unique considerations in the anaesthetic management of patients with diabetes mellitus. *Curr Opin Anaesthesiol* 1996; **9**: 245–6.

27 Raucoules-Aimé M, Grimaud D. Diabetes mellitus: implications for the anaesthesiologist. *Curr Opin Anaesthesiol* 1996; **9**: 247–53.

28 Anon. Drugs in the peri-operative period 2 – Corticosteroids and therapy for diabetes mellitus. *Drug Ther Bull* 1999; **37**: 68–70.

29 Alberti KGMM, Thomas DJB. The management of diabetes during surgery. *Br J Anaesth* 1979; **51**: 693–710.

30 Breivik H. Perianaesthetic management of patients with endocrine disease. *Acta Anaesthesiol Scand* 1996; **40**: 1004–15.

31 Roizen MF. Anesthetic implications of concurrent diseases. In: Miller RD, ed. *Anesthesia*, 4th edn. New York: Churchill Livingstone, 1994.

32 Sieber FE. Evaluation of the patient with endocrine disease or diabetes. In: Longnecker DE, Tinker JH, Morgan GE, eds. *Principles and Practice of Anesthesiology*, 2nd edn. St Louis: Mosby, 1998.

33 Stoelting RK. Preoperative management of the patient receiving glucocorticoids. *Curr Opin Anaesthesiol* 1997; **10**: 227–8.

34 Stenstrom G, Haljamae H, Tisell LE *et al.* Influence of preoperative treatment with phenoxybenzamine on the incidence of adverse cardiovascular reactions during anaesthesia and surgery for pheochromocytoma. *Acta Anaesthesiol Scand* 1985: **29**; 797.

130

35 Sterns RH. Severe symptomatic hyponatraemia: treatment and outcome. *Ann Intern Med* 1987; **107**: 656.

36 Fawcett WJ, Haxby EJ, Male DA. Magnesium: physiology and pharmacology. *Br J Anaesth* 1999; **83**: 302–20.

37 Engelhardt T, Webster NR. Pulmonary aspiration of gastric contents in anaesthesia. *Br J Anaesth* 1999; **83**: 453–60.

38 Pugh RNH, Murray-Lyon IM, Dawson JL *et al*. Transection of the oesophagus for bleeding oesophageal varices. *Br J Surg* 1973; **60**: 646–9.

39 Siefkin AD, Bolt RJ. Preoperative evaluation of the patient with gastrointestinal or liver disease. *Med Clin North Am* 1979; **63**: 1309.

40 Tobias MD. Evaluation of patients with hepatic disease. In: Longnecker DE, Tinker JH, Morgan GE, eds. *Principles and practice of anesthesiology*, 2nd edn. St Louis: Mosby, 1998: 334–59.

41 Brown Jr BR. Anaesthesia and liver disease. In: Nimmo WS, Rowbotham DJ, Smith G, eds. *Anaesthesia*, 2nd edn. Oxford: Blackwell Science, 1994.

42 Dawson JL. Jaundice and anoxic renal damage: protective effect of mannitol. *BMJ* 1964; **1**: 810–11.

43 Lauer A, Saccaggi A, Ronco C, Belledone M, Glabman S, Bosch JP. Continuous arteri-ovenous hemofiltration in the critically ill patient. *Ann Intern Med* 1983; **99**: 455–60.

44 Arroyo V, Gines P, Planas R *et al*. Management of patients with cirrhosis and ascites. *Semin Liver Dis* 1986; **6**: 353.

45 Miller RD. Current perspectives on blood transfusion. International Anesthesia Research Society 1990 Review course lectures, 57–61.

46 Carson JL, Poses RM, Spence RK, Bonavita G. Severity of anaemia and operative mortality and morbidity. *Lancet* 1988; **1**: 727–9.

47 Andrews CM, Lane DW, Bradley JG. Iron pre-load for major joint replacement. *Transfus Med* 1997; **7**: 281–6.

48 Practical guidelines for blood component therapy. A report by the American Society of Anesthesiologists task force on blood component therapy. *Anesthesiology* 1996; **84**: 732–47.

49 Vijay V, Cavenagh JD, Yate P. The anaesthetist's role in acute sickle cell crisis. *Br J Anaesth* 1998; **80**: 820–8.

50 Esseltine DW, Baxter MRN, Bevan JC. Sickle cell states and the anaesthetist. *Can J Anaesth* 1988; **35**: 385–403.

51 Bullingham A, Priestley M. Anaesthetic management of patients being treated with anti-coagulants. *Curr Opin Anaesthesiol* 1997; **10**: 234–39.

52 Bryan AJ, Butchart EG. Prosthetic heart valves and anticoagulant management during non-cardiac surgery. *Br J Surg* 1995; **82**: 577–8.

53 Vandermeulen EP, van Aken H, Vermylen J. Anticoagulants and spinal-epidural anes-thesia. *Anesth Analg* 1994; **79**: 1165–77.

54 Haljamäe H. Thromboprophylaxis, coagulation disorders, and regional anaesthesia. *Acta Anaesthesiol Scand* 1996; **40**: 1024–40.

55 Sonksen JR, Kong KL, Holder R. Magnitude and time course of impaired primary haemostasis after stopping chronic low and medium dose aspirin in healthy volunteers. *Br J Anaesth* 1999; **82**: 360–5.

56 Gill JC. Therapy of factor VIII deficiency. *Semin Thromb Hemostasis* 1993; **19**: 1–12.

57 Macik BG. Treatment of factor VIII inhibitors: products and strategies. *Semin Thromb Hemostasis* 1993; **19**: 13–24.

58 Mannuci PM. Desmopressin: a non transfusional form of treatment for congenital and acquired bleeding disorders. *Blood* 1988; **72**: 1449.

59 Eschbach JW, Egrie JC, Downing MR *et al*. Treatment of the anaemia of progressive renal failure with recombinant human erythropoietin. *N Engl J Med* 1989; **321**: 158.

60 DiMinno G. Platelet dysfunction in uremia: multifaceted defect partially corrected by dialysis. *Am J Med* 1985; **79**: 552.

61 Mannucci PM, Remuzzi G, Pusineri F *et al*. 1-Desamino-8-d-arginine vasopressin shortens the bleeding time in uremia. *N Engl J Med* 1983; **308**: 8.

62 Margolis DM, Saylor JL, Geisse G *et al*. Upper gastrointestinal disease in chronic renal failure: a prospective evaluation. *Arch Intern Med* 1978; **138**: 1214.

63 Gamulin Z, Forster A, Morel D *et al*. Effects of infrarenal aortic cross-clamping on renal hemodynamics in humans. *Anesthesiology* 1984; **61**: 394.

64 Yee J, Parasuraman R, Narins RG. Selective review of key perioperative renal-electrolyte disturbance in chronic renal failure patients. *Chest* 1999; **115**; 149S–157S.

65 Chui PT, Chung DCW. Medications to withhold or continue in the preoperative consultation. *Curr Anaesth Crit Care* 1998; **9**: 302–6.

66 Fee JPH, McCaughey W. Preoperative preparation, premedication and concurrent drug therapy. In: Nimmo WS, Rowbotham DJ, Smith G, eds. *Anaesthesia*, 2nd edn. Oxford: Blackwell Science, 1994.

67 Baraka A. Anaesthesia and myaesthenia gravis. *Can J Anaesth* 1992; **39**: 476–86.

68 Alley CT, Diedorf SF. Myaesthenia gravis and muscular dystrophies. *Curr Opin Anaesthesiol* 1997; **10**: 248–53.

69 Karan SM, Colonna-Romano P, Rosenberg H. Evaluation of the patient with neuromuscular disease. In: Longnecker DE, Tinker JH, Morgan GE, eds. *Principles and practice of anesthesiology*, 2nd edn. St Louis: Mosby, 1998.

7: Patient consent*

CHRISTOPHER HENEGHAN

Introduction

There must be consent for medical treatment. Medical treatment is intended to benefit the patient, not the doctor. The patient or, if relevant, someone on their behalf, must agree. This is a necessary consequence of the Common Law right to personal physical integrity. When no-one can give consent, other legal principles guide us.

We are required to get consent because to perform even a physical examination without consent would constitute an assault. Simply laying on hands without consent may be a tort, i.e. a breach of civil law giving rights to the victim, and a crime, i.e. a breach of criminal law incurring penalties for the perpetrator. Though likely damages for such minor assaults as examining an abdomen without the patient's consent would be negligible and assault would only attract criminal penalties if criminal intent could be proved, there is clearly a risk to professional status, as the General Medical Council (GMC) might well seek an explanation.

GMC interest would certainly be aroused in any criminal assault case and this seems to be being extended to include performing an operation not specifically approved, even when the procedure was traditionally covered by the form of consent actually given. It has been attempted to apply this to anaesthesia, breaking the anaesthetic down into components consented for and those not (see below), though so far this has not succeeded. However, there can be no doubt that boundaries are being pushed back and new ground being broken by the lawyers. When they fail to convince the judges, they refine their arguments until they succeed. We would be ill advised to be complacent about anything relating to medicolegal matters and to that end I always tell a patient when I intend to perform a procedure they might not have expected from general knowledge of anaesthesia (and if they have any

---

* Law changes: this chapter is up to date as of September 2000. The law discussed is that of England & Wales, though Scots and Northern Irish law of tort are effectively identical. Comments on foreign law are not authoritative. Application of law to specific cases should be the subject of independent legal advice.

Where 'he, him, his etc' appear in the text, they should be taken to refer to both sexes.

objections, discuss them). The more the viewpoints of the law and of the GMC move away from that of the doctor and towards that of the patient, however piously we might wish to be seen to support such moves, the more we have to watch the trends, and our backs, making sure we are still up to date on the reasons they might have for suing us.

Consent

Consent is the agreement by the patient (or another on their behalf; see below) to undergo a specified treatment or procedure. Its requirement is not restricted to operations, but covers physical examination, investigations, anaesthesia, and anything else where it is intended to breach a patient's personal physical integrity, albeit in their own interest. The doctor, or other person carrying out the procedure, may advise that a procedure should take place but cannot usually decide that it will. Only the patient, usually, can decide.

The right of the individual to control of their own bodily integrity underlies the rule that only a patient may consent. It is their body, they must decide what can be done to it. An individual has the right to refuse proposed treatment "for a good reason, a bad reason, or no reason at all".[1]*There are, however, limits to this seemingly sweeping statement (as when a patient is not of sound mind; see below). Though a patient may accept or refuse an offer of treatment, they may not insist on a different form of treatment which is not on offer. This might seem at first a meaningless quibble. However, suppose for example you are referred a patient whom you believe to be unfit for any form of anaesthesia save spinal. The patient is entitled to refuse spinal anaesthesia and, it seems to me, is entitled to have the consequences of such refusal explained. The patient is not entitled to insist on any other form of anaesthesia and the courts will not require you to administer any other form. Of course, the patient may be entitled to a second opinion and might be entitled to sue you if your failure to offer other forms of anaesthesia was negligent; if your decision would be supported by a responsible, respectable, reputable body of opinion in the specialty, the patient should lose.

It may seem, at times, that the patient has chosen their treatment, which seems inconsistent with the above. I would suggest this is the sort of occasion where a range of options has been put before the patient. The doctor is prepared to offer other treatments, perhaps less good in his or her opinion, but still reputable options. In such a case a patient may choose. Agreement has been reached and treatment follows. Where a patient insists on treatment not in the range of proper options, the scenario set out in the last paragraph unfolds.

---

* A refusal of consent to transfusion on religious grounds.

Withholding consent: communication

Consent may be withheld in advance. In a Canadian case,[2] it was held that a Jehovah's Witness card found on an unconscious accident victim, stating that no blood should be administered under any circumstances, was a valid restriction the doctor was not entitled to ignore. More widely, advance directives or living wills are documents that we are likely to be faced with in future. These are documents setting out, at a time when the individual is in possession of their mental faculties, forms of treatment which they withhold consent for at any time in the future when they are no longer in possession of their mental faculties. The GMC[3] advises that we must respect these documents, provided the withholding of consent is clearly applicable to the circumstances and there is no evidence that a patient has changed their mind. Though living wills have not yet been tested by the English courts, it seems probable that they would take the same line as the GMC and, in the absence of a contrary precedent, so should we.

Evidence of consent: forms and notes

What about consent forms? Does a patient have to sign one? And do they have to sign a separate one for the anaesthetic? This vexed question is simply answered. There is no legal requirement for a signed consent form before anaesthesia, surgery or any other procedure. A consent form is merely evidence that the patient has consented, at the time they signed it, to the procedure described (see, for example, Chatterton v Gerson).[4] Even that is to oversimplify, as the details of the procedure are not usually entered on the form, only its name, so it is possible to subdivide even this evidence into components. But evidence is all a consent form can be. Though it is written in a form superficially resembling a contract (two signatures, dates, etc.), it is not a contract* and does not bind the patient. They may change their mind about consent at any time up to the moment of anaesthesia, when it is no longer physically possible, and they may change their mind halfway through if they are having the procedure under local. The consent form has no impact on this right to withdraw consent.†

The persons on whom a consent form is binding are the doctors. We have consent and are protected from suit or prosecution in respect of what is

---

* For the legalistically inclined, the consent form is not a contract because there is no consideration and, of course, because it is not intended to be.
† If this seems like a legal quibble, as all the patient has to do is walk away, bear in mind that patients may be to an extent under the doctor's control – may even be physically restrained. In reality, of course, withdrawal of consent part way through must result in renegotiation and discussion, but what if the patient is sedated? Can consent given when unsedated be withdrawn when sedated? I do not think the courts have addressed this yet.

written on the form (as long as we have properly fulfilled requirements about information). In spite of the broad-brush wording of the standard form, we may not perform any other procedure unless it is genuinely necessary in an emergency. This does not extend to doing another procedure because it would be more convenient for the patient (or the doctor) to do it under the same anaesthetic, nor to doing something which was discussed but for which there was no clear consent. True emergencies should be thought of as where there would be serious risk to life or limb in waking the patient to acquire consent for a more extensive procedure.

A consent form being not legally binding on the patient has the consequence that it must be recent to be relevant evidence of consent. If it was signed in outpatients months or years before, it must clearly be confirmed.

A consent form is merely evidence of consent. What other forms of evidence might there be? There may be consent by compliance, where consent is implied by a patient allowing a procedure to be undertaken while they are awake. There may be problems with this, as for example a patient stating that they did not know what was planned until it began, once the procedure started they were afraid to move/ask questions/complain, and so on. Usually in such a case a patient would be expected to make something of the issue immediately afterwards and in such a case it would be advisable to note such a conversation.

There may be verbal consent, without a consent form. It may be explicitly noted or evidenced by implication. The latter is the usual route anaesthetists take to evidencing consent and it is unusual to note explicit consent. Usually there is only a record of the consultation. If any doubt is anticipated, it would be advisable explicitly to note consent and it seems indisputably good practice to record any refusal of consent, both as evidence and as an aide mémoire. It is of course open to a doctor, if it seems appropriate, to get a witness to countersign the record of consent in the notes.

Informed consent

A great deal has been written and said on this subject over the last 20 years. The cynical view is that this is a result of lawyers trying to win the unwinnable cases – where a recognised, non-negligent complication has ensued from some treatment – by saying that if the patient had known of the risk, they would not have consented. Legal argument has flowed around two principal concepts: doctor-centred and patient-centred standards. The first essentially looks at information doctors have regarded as appropriate to give to patients. This derives from the Bolam case[5] which set out that standards of care, and of information given to patients, were assessed on the basis of what a group of responsible, respectable, reputable (the words are used interchangeably) doctors, even if a minority, would support. This has been shortened to the "responsible minority test". The other variant centres around what a reasonable patient would regard as necessary information to allow them to come to a decision as to whether to have the proposed treatment. There have been variants on this and one of those variants has recently been adopted in Australia.[6] This idea has been called the "doctrine of informed consent" and it is the test used in some of the United States of America.*

Clearly, there is a potential difference between the two tests, especially in a society such as Britain where traditionally patients have not been expected to understand their treatment and where many still say such things as "I'm in your hands, doctor" when faced with an explanation. Further, some might argue that fully informed consent is impossible unless you are qualified in the relevant specialty and the whole concept of it negates the whole reason for having professions. If you must understand all the risks yourself, what are the doctors for? Nevertheless, it is also a reasonable argument that a patient who wants to know is entitled to.

The House of Lords was called upon to review this point in Sidaway,[7] a case involving paralysis after cervical spine surgery. In their judgement they tried to square the circle by saying, first, that informed consent forms no part of English law but second, that a patient should have enough information to make an informed decision. Third, if a doctor judges that to give full information might frighten a patient off accepting really necessary treatment, he or she should withhold that information but fourth, if a patient asks, we must answer truthfully.[†] Fifth, we should not withhold information of a substantial risk of grave adverse consequences (the example from a Canadian case[8] was a 10% risk of a stroke) and sixth, if the court thought we had blundered, it would be entitled to say so.

This bewildering array of options has been widely simplified to the concept that we must give patients enough information to allow them to make an informed choice. This engagingly circular, almost cosmetic, definition, though it has no strict legal basis on any judgement or statute, has come to be a standard form of words in government and other public documents. As such, it would certainly be defensible practice under the Bolam doctor-centred test to give patients enough information to allow them an informed choice; one can only hope that the courts will accept that enough was enough.

Interestingly, the GMC document referred to earlier[3] takes a considerably stronger line than this, insisting that we must tell patients basic information, even if they insist they do not want to know details. It also takes the line that "... you should not withhold relevant information unless you judge this would cause the patient serious harm..." and repeatedly uses the term "informed consent", but in a way which seems to mean "consent after giving sufficient information to make an informed decision". This is not,

* Though frequently asserted, it is not true that all American states use the informed consent test – it is not even a majority of states.
† They did not address the scenario of how to proceed if a patient asks for information, but we think they actually do *not* want to know.

obviously, a legal document, though once again to follow it would clearly give one a defence under Bolam.

So what should we actually tell patients? What is "enough information to allow them to make an informed choice"? Here we see the disadvantage of uncertainty in the law. Whether we have said enough will depend on a judge's interpretation of that phrase, assuming he finds it applies. My practice is to give a brief description of likely events and add more detail for anything patients might not be expected to anticipate (neck lines, postoperative intensive care, epidural, and so on), include "information of substantial risks of grave adverse consequences", if any, and allow the patient a period of "any questions". If there is room for choice about anaesthetic techniques, I always try as far as possible to accommodate patient wishes, if there is no significant bearing on safety. I certainly do not tell patients all basic information, nor tell them details they clearly do not want to know. Above all, I try to be sensitive to the patient and their apparent desires. I cannot tell you if that is enough nor, I think, can anyone else, until the courts are asked to test our different approaches.

The court has to an extent resolved this difficulty by adopting virtually the same line as the Australian courts, albeit so far only in the Court of Appeal, in Pearce v United Bristol Healthcare NHST [1999] PIQR 53. In a case of consent to opt for vaginal delivery rather than caesarean section, where the obstetrician omitted to warn of the slightly increased risk of stillbirth with vaginal delivery, it was held that doctors have a duty to inform the patient of a significant risk "if the information is needed so that the patient can determine for him or herself as to what course he or she should adopt". In deciding whether a risk is significant, the doctor will have to take into account "all the relevant considerations, which include the ability of the patient to comprehend what he has to say to him or her and the state of the patient at the particular time, both ... physical ... and ... emotional ...". If approved by the House of Lords, we will have moved from the position of no informed consent in English Law to that where any relevant information must be transmitted: 200-page consent forms cannot be far away!

Sectionalised consent

What of gaining consent, say, for a caudal as an analgesic addendum to a general anaesthetic? Or for insertion of analgesic suppositories for postoperative analgesia? Authorities differ on this. On the one hand there is a first-instance (i.e. lower court) decision,[9] not (as far as I know) approved in an appeal court, that a procedure cannot be sectionalised. If you divide up consent for different parts of the anaesthetic, you could also divide up consent for bits of the operation. If consent is given for local, regional or general anaesthesia, as here, then it cannot be sectionalised. I suspect the judge was unduly influenced by expert evidence that when the 1987 case occurred, they would not have sought consent for such parts of a procedure (though they would have done in 1992). Certainly, this decision is dubious (in part because it is based on the judicially much deplored tort of Battery rather than Negligence) as it seems to run counter to the general development of the law and has been seriously doubted by one eminent commentator.[10] It would probably be dangerous to rely on.

Modern practice leans toward warning of anything a patient might be aware of in the postoperative period, as is demonstrated by the GMC's decision[11] to admonish an anaesthetist who inserted, without prior discussion, a Voltarol suppository (in the event inadvertently into the vagina) after an outpatient tooth extraction. Those anaesthetists who were outraged by this decision, not least because there is no appeal from a mere admonition from the GMC, might reflect that it *is* in line with the direction of development of medical law and that this approach is likely to find favour with the courts.

Mental incapacity

Patients not capable of making decisions for themselves, or potentially not so capable, seem to me to fall into three categories: the unconscious, those with "learning difficulties" or for other reasons temporarily or permanently mentally incompetent, and children.

Unconscious patients

Unconscious patients and other "incompetent" adults – those unable to give consent – have long been a source of confusion, still extant in some quarters. There has been a practice, perhaps based on the misconception that there *must* be a signed consent form, of getting relatives to sign a consent form "on behalf" of the unconscious. This has, on occasion, ludicrously been extended to professional carers, neighbours or any desperate surrogate for a next of kin available. The law is now clear that this is not the right route. *No individual may give consent for physical treatment for physical illness on behalf of another adult.*[12]

What do we do about it, then? No-one can give consent so how do we proceed? Clearly, we must be contemplating emergency or urgent procedures or we would wait until the patient regained their reasoning powers. In these circumstances, the law requires us to *act in the patient's best interests*, taking into account our knowledge of the patient and any known views, whether through information from relatives, carers or others or through advance directives/living wills (and of course noting all these matters fully in the records).* If there is

---

* The Diane Blood case, much reported in the press (R v Human Fertilisation & Embryology Authority, Ex P Blood [1997] 2WLR 806 (CA)), seems to contradict this, in that the applicant was eventually allowed to be fertilised with sperm drawn from her deceased husband without his consent before his death. In the judgement, it was held that though the acquisition and storage of the sperm *was* unlawful, there was no right to prevent its use abroad. The law is therefore unchanged.

doubt, and particularly when dealing with non-urgent treatment decisions (such as withdrawal of treatment in persistent vegetative state), it may be necessary to seek further medical opinions or to apply to the courts.

Usually there is no doubt and decisions are straightforward. We must of course consult relatives to ascertain the patient's views, if any, and this, perhaps, is the modern version of surrogate signatories to the consent form. Certainly, there can be no doubt that the fullest discussion with relatives, taking them along with you in any decision making, can save a great deal of problems later.[†] However, whatever the appearances, the relatives do not give permission for treatment or its withdrawal: the law requires *us*, as doctors, to make these decisions in the best interests of the patient. Further, it is clear that those best interests may include discontinuation of futile treatment.[13] Of course, the situation must be handled sensitively, especially when considering withdrawing or not offering futile treatment, and if appropriate, there should be recourse to second opinions and time for reflection. In the final analysis, however, such decisions cannot be ducked.

On occasion, there is dispute among the relatives as to a patient's view on forms of treatment (as in, for example, Re T[1]). Such disputes may be soluble by proper explanation, perhaps supported by second opinion: recourse to the courts might, however, be necessary (see, for example, Re G, unreported[14]).

Incompetent adults

The deeply unconscious represent one problem, with its own solutions, but there is no doubt as to a patient's current mental incapacity. What about those with "learning difficulties" or perhaps severe Alzheimer's disease? What do we do about a clearly demented patient who needs anaesthesia for fractured neck of femur? And does it make a difference whether this patient refuses the operation?

There has been a run of cases in this area. The basic rule is the same as for the unconscious: act in the patient's best interests, guided, where appropriate, by knowledge of their wishes. This again may be a matter for advance directives and/or communication with kin. What if the treatment proposed is not clearly in their best interests? Sterilisation in fertile females has come up repeatedly, as has hysterectomy and abortion. It has been usual to apply to the courts for consent, though the court may refuse to make a declaration if it sees the treatment as obviously necessary.

Under the Mental Health Act, there are statutory exceptions relating to treatment for mental illness. In a recent case[15] relating to depression in a late pregnancy, where consent for caesarean section for preeclampsia was refused, permission for caesarean section was given by a court under

---

[†]How this accords with our duty of confidentiality to the patient seems as yet unresolved. Pragmatically, however, or cynically, one can do worse than to bear in mind that when a patient dies, it is their heirs who can sue.

Mental Health Act provisions. This was set aside on appeal (though after the caesarean) and recommendations relating to how to take such a case through the courts were made. In particular, both parties must be represented at any hearing (the patient, if "unable to instruct solicitors", should be represented through the official solicitors) and all the facts must be available to the court. In another case, also a pregnancy case, where the mother had paranoid schizophrenia, it was held that there can be physical treatment for mental illness under the Mental Health Act,[16] but this area is dubious enough, in my view, to suggest a need at very least for counsel's opinion before embarking on intervention.*

What of cases where there is doubt about mental capacity, and competence to decide? This was addressed in the remarkable case of Re C.[17] C was a 68-year-old paranoid schizophrenic, confined to Broadmoor and suffering from delusions, including that he had an international medical practice. He sought an injunction to prevent a hospital amputating his leg in the event of gangrene in it recurring. The court applied the statement in Re T[1] that treatment may be refused for a good reason, a bad reason or no reason at all, as long as the individual was competent to make the decision, and then went on to give the test of competence. This has three stages, as follows.

1. The patient must be able to comprehend and retain information about the procedure.
2. He must believe this information.
3. Weighing that information, balancing risks and needs, he arrives at a choice.

Though this seems a cumbersome procedure for assessment of competence, it seems an appropriate solution to the problem of how to assess mental competence without being influenced by the actual choice made. This test is now standard.

Finally, what of the Alzheimer's patient refusing repair of fractured neck or femur, an all too common problem? May we anaesthetise him? It seems to me that we should apply the Re C[17] test set out above and I would expect that most such patients would fail at the first step, not being able either to comprehend or to retain the information about the procedure, and probably the third as well. In such a circumstance, we would be required to act in his best interests, taking into account any known views, just as for any other patient who is not competent to decide.

---

* It may be that these cases will mark the end of attempts to enforce caesarean section on women who refuse it. Whatever one's opinion on what the law should be – and it is unlikely to change in the present climate – it now seems clear that it is no different for pregnant women: if mentally competent (see later), they can refuse caesarean section for a good reason, a bad reason or no reason at all. This perhaps brings to a close a run of none too happy cases originating with enforced caesareans on black women in pre-second World War America, though no doubt the debate will continue until the fetus has equal rights to the mother.

Premedication

It is a surprisingly common occurrence to be presented with a previously competent patient who has received a premedicant sedative but has not yet signed their consent form. What do we do about that? The simple response is that they cannot give consent under the influence of a premedicant. This approach must be commended for its caution, though it may be overcautious to cover all cases. What if this approach means that the operation will be postponed for several weeks/months/years? It must not be forgotten that the consent form is only evidence of consent, not the consent itself. Thus if a patient has clearly consented to the proposed treatment throughout a series of encounters with medical staff and there is no doubt about the proposed procedure, it may be acceptable to proceed. If, however, there is any doubt, for example as to side or digit, or as to extent of the procedure, it is clear that it may be incorrect to attempt to resolve that doubt with the patient premedicated. Though it might be tempting to try to apply the test of mental competence outlined previously to this situation, I think that this would be risky and I would not recommend it.

Children

Parents may consent on behalf of their children, as may legal guardians. No difficulty there. Who else may consent? The child, the court, the local authority for children in care. Yes to all of those questions, in certain circumstances.

By statute, a child of 16 or over may consent for their own treatment,[18] unless they are not competent (on the Re C[17] test), when parents, guardians or the court may consent on their behalf or, failing all of these, we must act in their best interests, as for all other patients. A younger child may consent if "Gillick[19] competent", where they have "sufficient intelligence and understanding to appreciate fully what is proposed"* (the case related to prescription of contraceptives to under-age girls). A local authority may also consent on behalf of a child in care and a court for any child even if over 16 (see below).

What if parents withhold consent for urgent treatment, and there is no time to apply to a court? For example, a child road traffic accident (RTA) victim needing blood transfusion, whose parents are Jehovah's Witnesses. Must we apply to the court, even though the child will bleed to death long before the process is complete? I have been unable to find a legal precedent directly on this point, but the GMC's leaflet on consent[3] contains the following statement:

---

* One wonders whether if Gillick[19] came up now, the courts would use the test in Re C[17].

In an emergency where you consider it is in the child's best interests to proceed, you may treat the child, provided it is limited to that treatment which is reasonably required in that emergency.

This is consistent with the course of action required in adult cases, that in the absence of consent, and in cases of necessity, we must act in the patient's best interests. The parental refusal of consent should be seen, as in Re W[20] (see below), not as a weapon to be used against us but as the absence of one particular shield: the common law defence of necessity has to be our shield in the absence of specific consent.

Who may withhold consent? Nobody, if a person entitled to give consent has given it. Thus, in Re W,[20] a 16-year-old girl, who under Family Law Reform Act 1969[18] could consent, who was Gillick competent to consent as found by the judge, refused treatment for anorexia nervosa. The Court of Appeal said:

- it had the power to override that refusal of consent
- that this inherent jurisdiction was exercisable in respect of any child, whether a ward of court or not
- that the Family Law Reform Act[18] gave a right to consent but not to withhold consent
- that "...no minor of whatever age has power by refusing consent to treatment to override a consent to treatment by someone who has parental responsibility for a minor and a *fortiori** a consent by a court...".

Consent on behalf of a child is a shield for the doctors and whoever gives it confers that shield: it cannot be withdrawn, even by the patient. The court should take into account the child's best interests and parental views, but the jurisdiction remains. Interestingly, when a similar case to Re W[20], relating to a heart transplant, reached the courts in summer 1999, the child patient from Re W[20] was reported as being very grateful for having her refusal to consent overridden by the Court, as she now saw it as mistaken.

It would seem, therefore, that though there are paediatric anaesthetists who refuse to hold down a child for induction even at a very young age, *bona fide* parental consent would protect us when we undertake such an action.

Surgery

Who is responsible for ensuring that the right operation gets done? The operating surgeon, the house surgeon, the anaesthetising anaesthetist, another anaesthetist who saw the patient on the ward, the scrub nurse, the theatre receptionist, the ward nurse, the operating department assistant

---

*=therefore more strongly

(ODA), the theatre orderly? It is probably safe to rule out the orderly, the ODA and the receptionist (unless they are a nurse) but what of the others? The question arises because all these people, at some time or another, may involve themselves in checking consent forms, theatre lists, etc. It produces the curious scenario of a scrub nurse refusing to hand the sterilising swab to the surgeon until the nurse has checked the consent form personally.

Whilst I am a firm advocate of everyone checking up on everyone else as much as seems appropriate, because we all make mistakes, I doubt whether anyone but the surgeon actually has legal liability for doing the correct operation. In the NHS, where we are all employees of the hospital we work in, this is a quibble, as the hospital is vicariously liable for all our actions and it is a purely internal matter how liability is divided up. Outside the health service, it might be different, with a hospital trying to shift the load onto one of the consultants to save itself – or its insurers – some money. There must be an answer.

Though I know of no case directly to this point, it seems to me that the decision must depend on the facts of the case. Though the surgeon must be responsible in all cases, there may be odd circumstances, such as changes in the order of the list which the surgeon is not informed of, where that responsibility may be diluted. Thus it must be acceptable for a hospital to set up a system whereby the consent is checked by everyone through whose hands the patient passes, if only to protect itself. However, it cannot be denied that the actual acquiring of consent for surgery is the responsibility of the surgical team and ultimately the operating surgeon. Anaesthetists, scrub nurses, and others need to know what is planned, to plan their work accordingly, and need to keep everyone affected informed of any changes we initiate. However, the surgeon must know what he (or she) is doing, what he has discussed with the patient and what alternatives have been discussed. Often he is the only one who knows what operation he is actually doing while he is doing it. No-one else can seriously be thought to take on the ultimate responsibility for getting the consent and doing the right operation.

Conclusion

The law on consent may seem very confusing. There are several inconsistencies and apparent anomalies, not least as a result of court judgements such as Sidaway.[7] However, recent cases have clarified the position about consent on behalf of the unconscious and those of dubious mental competence, providing a tool for testing such competence, which has clarified consent on behalf of children and clarified withholding of consent in such cases. Though there is as yet no case law, advance directives/living wills seem to be coalescing into practical documents. However, there is still doubt about "sectionalised consent" and "informed consent", in spite of the adoption of a standard format by official documents, remains uncertain.

Whether the last item can be resolved completely until there has been a social sea change remains to be seen.

Decision plan

A decision plan to allow a rational, and legal, approach to consent in all cases is given below.

PATIENT CONSENT DECISION CHART

(Start at Competent Adults, and follow directions)

COMPETENT ADULTS

1. Is patient 18 years or over? If **NO**, go to "Children".

   YES

2. Is patient of sound mind? If **NO**, or in doubt, go to "Competence in Adults".

   YES

3. Does patient consent?　　If **NO**, (i) Do **NOT** proceed*, and
   　　　　　　　　　　　　　　　(ii) Consider whether this
   　　　　　　　　　　　　　　　　　brings competence into
   　　　　　　　　　　　　　　　　　question.
   　　　　　　　　　　　　　　If **YES** to (ii), go to
   　　　　　　　　　　　　　　　"Competence in Adults".

   YES – Record evidence if appropriate/ Consent Form, and proceed with procedure.

---

* Re T (Adult: Refusal of Treatment) [1992] 3WLR 782

145

COMPETENCE IN ADULTS

4. Is patient conscious and coherent? If **NO**, go to "Incompetent Adults".

YES

5. Apply Re C* test:
    Can patient comprehend **and** retain information about procedure?
    Does patient **believe** that information?
    Can patient weigh information and balance risks to arrive at a choice?

If **YES** to **all 3 steps** patient is competent **whatever his choice:** go to Q3 above.

If **NO** to any of steps in Q5, go to "Incompetent Adults".

INCOMPETENT ADULTS†

6. Is planned procedure **clearly** in patient's best interests (e.g. life saving, pain reducing)?
    If **NO**, do **NOT** proceed, and consider 2nd opinion, application to court, etc.

YES

7. Is there any **reason not to proceed** (advance directive/living will; knowledge of patient's views on proposed treatment from relatives)?
    If **YES**, do **NOT** proceed. Consider investigating further if time available.
    If **genuinely uncertain** (e.g. conflicting reports from relatives) consider application to courts if time allows.
If **NO** reason not to proceed, go to Q8.

8. Is procedure obviously necessary (urgent, fixation fractures, etc.)?

If **YES**, proceed with planned procedure: no other consent is necessary.

If **in doubt** (e.g. sterilisation, termination, nasogastric feeding in persistent vegetative state, etc.), consider application to courts.

---

* Re C (Refusal of Medical Treatment) [1994] 1FLR 31
† In Re F [1989] 1Med LR. 58

146

CHILDREN

9. Is child 16 or over* and competent (Re C[†] test)?
                                    If **NO**, go to Q11.

YES

10. Does child consent?   If **NO**, go to Q13.

YES – Record/Consent Form as appropriate, and proceed with procedure.

11. Is child "Gillick[‡] competent"(has he sufficient intelligence and under-standing to appreciate fully what is proposed)? If **NO**, go to Q13.

YES

12. Does child consent?   If **NO**, go to Q13.

YES – Record/Consent Form as appropriate, and proceed with procedure.

13. Is there a person who can give consent? This may be parent, legal guardian, local authority (for children in care), court.[§]
                        If **NO**, is procedure obviously necessary
                        (life saving, fixation fractures, etc.)?
                        If **YES**, proceed with planned procedure:
                        no other consent is necessary.**
                        If **in doubt** wait until parent/guardian
                        available obtain second opinion or apply to
                        court, as appropriate.

YES

14. Does that person give consent?   If **NO**, 14.1 is procedure obviously necessary (life saving, fixation fractures, etc.)?
                                      If **YES**, proceed with planned procedure: no other consent is necessary.**
                                      If **NO** wait until other parent/ guardian available or apply to court, as appropriate.

YES – Record/Consent Form as appropriate, and proceed with procedure.[††]

---

* Family Law Reform Act 1969, s8
† Re C (Refusal of Medical Treatment) [1994] 1FLR 31
‡ Gillick v Norfolk & W Wisbech AHA [1986] AC112
§ Re W (a minor) (Medical Treatment) [1992] 4All ER 627
** In Re F [1989] 1Med LR. 58
†† Re W (a minor) (Medical Treatment) [1992] 4All ER 627

1   Re T (Adult: Refusal of Treatment) [1992] 3WLR 782 (CA); confirmed Airedale[13].
2   Malette v Shulman et al [1991] 2Med LR. 162–168 (Ont. CA).
3   *Seeking patients' consent: the ethical considerations.* London: GMC, 1999.
4   Chatterton v Gerson [1981] 1All ER 257.
5   Bolam v Friern HMC [1957] 1WLR 582.
6   Rogers v Whittaker [1993] 4Med LR 79 (HC Aus).
7   Sidaway v Board of Governors of Bethlehem Royal Hospital [1985] AC 871 (HL).
8   Reibl v Hughes (1980) 114 DLR (3d) 1.
9   Davis v Barking, Havering & Brentwood HA [1993] 4Med LR 85 (QBD).
10 Grubb A. Commentary (1993) 1Med LRev. 389.
11 Unreported; see *BMJ*. 1995; **310**: 43–8.
12 In Re F [1989] 1Med LR 58 (HL).
13 Airedale NHST v Bland [1993] 4 Med LR: 39 (HL).
14 Grubb A. Commentary (1995) 3Med LRev 80.
15 St George's Healthcare NHS Trust v S.; R v Collins et al, ex P S [1998] 3All ER 673 (CA).
16 Tameside & Glossop Acute Services Trust v CH [1996] 1FLR 762.
17 Re C (Refusal of Medical Treatment) [1994] 1FLR 31.
18 Family Law Reform Act 1969, s8.
19 Gillick v Norfolk & W Wisbech AHA [1986] AC112.
20 Re W (a minor) (Medical Treatment) [1992] 4All ER 627.

8: Preoperative fasting

SARAH YOUNG, STEPHANIE PHILLIPS

Preoperative fasting allows time for gastric emptying, thus minimising the gastric residual volume. This should reduce the risk of regurgitation of gastric contents and subsequently the risk of aspiration of those contents into the lungs. This can lead to laryngeal spasm, respiratory obstruction, chemical pneumonitis, and potentially death. This chapter will review the reasons for preoperative fasting, outline normal gastric physiology and review the pathophysiology which may affect it. It will also outline the current international guidelines for preventing perioperative pulmonary aspiration as well as strategies for minimising the severity of aspiration should it occur.

History

In 1847, Snow observed that patients who had eaten prior to surgery often regurgitated during anaesthesia and in 1858 recommended that operations should be performed "about the time when a patient would be ready for another meal".[1,2] Patients were encouraged to partake of beef or China tea or glucose water up until three hours before elective surgery, possibly to provide calories to sustain them through the procedure and aid recovery.[3]

The first documented anaesthetic death in 1848 was due to aspiration. A 15-year-old girl undergoing extraction of a toenail under chloroform was described thus: "Her lips which had previously been of good colour, became suddenly blanched, and she sputtered slightly at the mouth as one in epilepsy". Her physician administered water and brandy which appeared to revive her. Later he gave more brandy, but "she rattled in her throat" and soon died. Initially her death was blamed on the anaesthetic. However, Simpson suggested that the water and brandy "were, of course allowed to rest in and fill up the pharynx of the patient and she choked or asphyxiated by the means that intended to give her life".[4]

Snow's guidelines were followed until 1946 when the obstetrician Mendelson described two distinct syndromes in a large retrospective review of 44 016 parturients undergoing general anaesthesia for vaginal and operative deliveries. In the first group, five women inhaled solid food leading to complete airway obstruction during anaesthesia. Three died and the other two suffered massive atelectasis. In the second group, 40 women aspirated liquid gastric contents and developed dyspnoea, cyanosis, and tachycardia. All remained afebrile and recovered completely. Mendelson went on to demonstrate the different pathophysiology of the two syndromes in an elegant set of rabbit experiments. He showed that in the first syndrome, the extent of the airway obstruction was determined by the size and shape of the particles and not the volume and pH of the aspirate. He then demonstrated that the second syndrome was due to acid aspiration, its severity being dependent on the increasing acidity of the gastric contents. If the pH was above 2.5 the lung changes were no different from those caused by water alone and the severity of lung injury increased as pH fell below 2.4. Mendelson completed his paper by suggesting various methods to minimise the incidence of aspiration associated with parturition. The suggestions he made, which are still relevant today, were: fasting women during labour, the use of regional anaesthetic techniques where possible, the use of agents to alkalinise and empty the stomach, and, most importantly, the availability of suitable equipment and trained medical personnel to administer the anaesthetic.[5,6]

Physiology and pathophysiology

Knowledge of the physiology of gastric emptying is needed to help understand the procedures undertaken to enhance the emptying of the full stomach and prevent aspiration. Beaumont in 1833, whilst observing Alexis St Martin, a man who had been left with a gastric fistula following a gunshot wound to the stomach, noted that a duration of five hours was necessary for the digestion of solid food into chyme and its passage through the pylorus.[7] Clear fluids were emptied "soon after they were received". These observations have been proved reliable and modern physiology holds that liquids empty under the control of the proximal stomach at a rate related to the gastroduodenal pressure gradient with a half-time of 12 minutes.[8]

Solids are firstly digested into liquid chyme and then emptied into the duodenum with 50% of the meal remaining in the stomach after two hours. Increasing acidity, osmolarity, and fatty acid content all delay the rate of normal gastric emptying. Normal gastric emptying is also influenced by many other factors such as drugs (opiates, alcohol, anticholinergics), high sympathetic tone due to pain or anxiety, mechanical outlet obstructions, and neuropathies, for example diabetes.[8-10]

Regurgitation occurs when gastric contents flow passively into the oesophagus. Aspiration occurs when the gastric contents pass via the pharynx and larynx to enter the lungs. Gastro–oesophageal reflux is normally prevented by the lower oesophageal sphincter, an indistinct area of high pressure at the lower end of the oesophagus. The oblique entry of the oesophagus into the stomach via the diaphragmatic hiatus acts as a valve, helping prevent reflux. Gastric volumes of 8–14 ml/kg are required to

overcome a competent lower oesophageal sphincter, indicating the distensi-
bility of the stomach and effectiveness of the sphincter.[11] Most patients have
a fasting residual gastric volume of about 100 ml and, assuming a normal
lower oesophageal sphincter, are at a low risk of reflux.[12] When the function
of the sphincter is compromised, as in a hiatus hernia, or when there is a
marked rise in the intragastric pressure (such as large intraabdominal mass,
gastric outflow or advanced bowel obstruction, use of suxamethonium,
Trendelenburg or prone position), reflux occurs which may then lead to
aspiration.

Many workers have attempted to characterise the nature of the aspirate
that leads to pathological pulmonary changes. Mendelson had already
demonstrated the importance of pH. Bosomworth and Hamelberg showed
that the addition of pepsin and gastrin to gastric acid had no additional
effects.[13] The volume of gastric contents with a pH below 2.5 needed to
cause significant pulmonary damage has still not been fully elucidated and,
due to ethical limitations, may never be. Different authors have quoted
various figures ranging between 0.4 ml/kg,[14] 1 ml/kg,[15] and 2 ml/kg.[16] More
recently, Raidoo reported that in monkeys, inhalation of 1 ml/kg of fluid
with a pH of 1 had a mortality of 50%.[17] The volume of gastric fluid with a
pH below 2.5 necessary to produce serious sequelae remains unknown.
Workers in this field often have to accept the definition of "at risk" to be
those with a residual gastric volume of over 25ml (0.4 ml/kg) and a pH
below 2.5.[14] Included in this at-risk population are up to 60% of adults,
76% of children, 75% of obese patients and between 27–73% of pregnant
patients.[12]

It is important to realise that aspiration is not an inevitable consequence
of reflux and that should aspiration occur it is unlikely the entire residual
gastric volume would be inhaled. No adult study has shown a correlation
between the development of postoperative pulmonary morbidity, the
volume of gastric contents and gastrooesphageal reflux.[12,18]

In summary, minimising the residual gastric volume may reduce the risk
of oesophageal reflux and subsequently pulmonary aspiration of gastric
contents. Aspiration, in turn, may lead to laryngeal spasm, chemical pneumonitis (small volume, low pH), near drowning (large volume, neutral pH),
and complete or partial respiratory obstruction due to particulate matter.
Any of these events can be life threatening. Many risk factors for reflux and
aspiration can be identified preoperatively, allowing the anaesthetist time
for adequate preparation of the patient, including selection of an appropriate fasting time and most suitable anaesthetic technique.

The normal population

The incidence of aspiration following clinically observed gastro–
oesophageal reflux is low. Olsson and colleagues report a figure of 1 per

2131 anaesthetics,[18] whilst Warner and colleagues report a figure of 1 per 3216 patients.[19] In Olsson's series the incidence of pulmonary morbidity following aspiration confirmed by radiological changes, so-called "aspiration pneumonitis", was 1 per 4521 patients. Most large series are retrospective and may be subject to underreporting. In everyday practice it appears that aspiration may occur more frequently than these authors suggest. However, the mortality rates remain low at 0.2 per 10 000 (1 per 50 000).[18] The majority of patients recover with appropriate treatment and have minimal long-term sequelae.[18,19]

In the fit, healthy adult with no known risk factors for regurgitation or aspiration (see below), the traditional fasting regimen of 6–8 hour abstinence from all oral intake has recently been questioned.[20,21] A number of studies have shown that drinking clear fluids until two hours preoperatively makes no significant difference to the residual volume or pH of gastric contents. Volumes of up to 1200 ml have been given and no adverse consequences reported.[22,23]

Few studies have considered the effect of reducing the duration of the solid fast. However, the risk of aspiration of particulate matter remains a concern. If the duration of the fluid fast is reduced, then food intake becomes less important.

The effect of premedication on gastric contents in otherwise fit and healthy patients has been studied. It has been shown that a single dose of an opiate given to this population has no effect on gastric volume or acidity.[24] Similarly anticholinergics such as atropine, hyoscine, and glycopyrrolate have little clinical effect when administered in normal doses.

Fasting guidelines are changing, not because they offer additional safety to the patient with regards to the risks of regurgitation and aspiration, but because there is no added benefit from the prolonged fluid fast. Potential advantages, such as patients reporting feeling significantly less thirsty and more satisfied compared to prior anaesthetics when offered fluids within 2–3 hours of surgery, have encouraged the more liberal approach.[25]

Prolonged fasting may also have disadvantages, leading to dehydration, hypoglycaemia, poor compliance, malaise and irritability, and increased stress levels. Despite the intentions of the patients' medical attendants, prolonged fasting often occurs in all age groups. There are many, often poor, reasons to explain why this may occur. Failure to follow or understand instructions means that on a morning list, despite fasting instructions stating "clear fluids up to four hours preoperatively", many children go to bed, sleep through the night and arrive in hospital already fasted for up to 12 hours.[26] Nil-by-mouth orders are often instituted long before the scheduled time of surgery to comply with ward protocol or convenience. Operating times are unpredictable and unexpected changes to schedules are frequent. Other preoperative preparations can exacerbate the problem such as the institution of clear fluid regimens and bowel preparations prior to abdominal surgery. Despite encouragement to drink, these patients may be nauseated, anorexic and often dehydrated. Patients who do not receive intravenous fluids intraoperatively effectively fast until the resumption of oral intake after surgery. This period may also be prolonged and contribute to further dehydration, headache, nausea, malaise, and reduced well-being. These effects are more significant in children, due to their smaller size and high metabolic rates, and the elderly because of their reduced ability to cope with physiological changes, as well as those with hypercoagulability and polycythaemia.[27]

Hypoglycaemia is perhaps the most feared complication of the prolonged fast and may occur in younger children. Conflicting evidence has emerged over the years regarding the incidence of hypoglycaemia induced by preoperative fasting which is defined as a blood glucose concentration of less than 2.2 mmol/l in the term neonate and less than 1.1 mmol/l in small and preterm babies.[28] An explanation for the differing results is that there may be a diurnal variation in metabolism. One study showed that despite a longer fast, patients on the morning lists had higher blood glucose levels than those scheduled later in the day. No child was found to be hypoglycaemic.[29] In another study, Thomas found that 28% of children who had fasted from 06.00 hours for an afternoon operation had blood glucose concentration less than 2.2 mmol/l. This compared with 0% in a group fed 10 ml/kg of milk four hours before the operation.[30] In this and other studies, age less than two years and weight below the third centile increased the likelihood of hypoglycaemia.[31]

It is known that only 50% of patients comply with doctors' prescribing instructions. It has been presumed that compliance with preoperative fasting instructions may also be a problem.[28] Education of the patient on the reasons for preoperative fasting, the nature of solids and clear fluids, and written as well as verbal instructions may improve compliance and safety. Despite the concerns of some workers that non-compliance may increase following the liberalisation in clear fluid intake, studies have failed to confirm this view.[32]

Malaise, irritability, and stress in the pre- and postoperative period have been linked to the effect of witholding fluids.[32] Patients allowed to drink until closer to their scheduled operation time report a better recovery than when fasted for prolonged periods.[33] In a survey of patients undergoing stressful preoperative procedures it was shown that the witholding of fluids rated second only to the stress of waiting for surgery. Allowing fluids until two hours preoperatively reduced anxiety levels in a study of adult patients.[34,35]

Current wisdom would recommend the avoidance of all solid food and fluids containing fats for at least six hours before induction of anaesthesia and allowing unlimited clear fluids until two hours prior to induction. Individual practitioners may choose to instruct patients to adhere to a longer fast to increase the certainty of an adequate time for gastric emptying, should unexpected changes occur to the operating schedule.

Patients at increased risk of aspiration

The risk factors for regurgitation or aspiration are outlined in Box 8.1. Patients in whom gastric emptying may be impaired or those at risk of gastrooesophageal reflux for other reasons must be considered individually. Many patients have several contributing factors that place them at increased risk of regurgitating as well as having increased residual gastric volume. The majority of these patients should be identified preoperatively, allowing the anaesthetist to formulate a management plan encompassing an adequate preoperative fasting time, pharmacological modification of the gastric contents and selection of an appropriate anaesthetic technique.

The pregnant patient

Pregnant women have delayed gastric emptying and potentially increased gastric volumes for several reasons. The gravid uterus alters the orientation

Box 8.1 Patients at increased risk of perioperative aspiration of gastric contents

Abnormal lower oesophageal sphincter
   Hiatus hernia (or symptoms of hiatus hernia)
   Pregnancy
   Children
   Oesophageal achalasia
Increased gastric volume/pressure
   Children
   Recent ingestion of food or fluids
   Large abdominal mass
   Obesity
   Pregnancy
   Suxamethonium
   Surgical position of the patient, e.g. Trendelenburg, prone or lithotomy
Delayed gastric emptying
   Recent trauma
   Bowel obstruction, ileus
   Autonomic neuropathy
   Drugs, including alcohol, opiates, anticholinergics
   Pregnancy
Potential airway problems
   Children
   Obese
   Pregnancy
   Reduced conscious level
   Abnormal airway anatomy

of the stomach, increasing intragastric pressure as well as reducing the efficacy of the lower oesophageal sphincter. Raised gastrin levels increase the rate of gastric secretion, higher progesterone levels relax the lower oesophageal sphincter and lower levels of motilin reduce gastric emptying. Although studies have not been consistent in showing an increase of volume or pH during various stages of pregnancy, the mechanical factors alone place these patients at high risk of regurgitation during anaesthesia. The risks of aspiration are further increased by multiple factors such as glottic oedema, large breasts, full dentition, need for the left lateral tilt position to displace the gravid uterus which combine to make intubation more difficult and fail more often.[24,36]

Current teaching holds that after the 16th week of gestation, patients should undertake a minimum six-hour fast for both fluids and solids, routinely receive preoperative antacids and H_2 blockers and a rapid-sequence induction should be used if general anaesthesia becomes necessary. Once painful contractions are established, oral intake is restricted to clear fluids.[37] A recent study confirms the risks incurred by allowing women a light diet during labour. Residual gastric volumes were significantly higher and vomiting was 20% more frequent in study patients compared to demographically matched controls.[38] There is no consensus regarding the correct anaesthetic management of the postpartum patient and evidence as to when gastric emptying returns to normal is conflicting. In the early postpartum period it is safest to manage the woman as if she was still pregnant as the residual effects of pregnancy hormones, drugs, and endogenous catecholamines released in response to pain, blood loss, and anxiety may still be influencing the rate of gastric emptying.[37]

The obese patient

The obese patient is at increased risk of silent regurgitation and aspiration. The weight of the abdominal contents interferes with gastric emptying as well as the function of the lower oesophageal sphincter, leading to an increased residual gastric volume. However, one review of the literature actually opposes this view, suggesting that obese patients are at no greater risk of regurgitation and aspiration than the lean and may in fact have more rapid gastric emptying. When looking at unpremedicated, non-diabetic obese patients who are free from gastrooesophageal pathology, it was found that they were less likely to have high volume and low pH residual gastric volume than lean patients; however, these findings did not reach statistical significance. The fact that patients with a history of gastrooesophageal disease were excluded may have biased this finding as they are often clinically symptomatic of reflux and peptic ulcer disease.[39]

Obese patients have a higher incidence of difficulty in airway management with resultant gastric distension and reflux.[40] Latent autonomic neuropathy due to diabetes mellitus may also contribute to delayed gastric emptying.[8] Patient positioning is more difficult and rapid turning of the patient into the lateral position to minimise aspiration may simply not be possible.

As obese patients are at a higher risk of reflux and aspiration from multiple pathologies, all aspects of their preoperative care need to be planned. Gastro–oesophageal disease, delayed gastric emptying and potential airway management problems make adequate preoperative preparation essential. Weight loss prior to surgery, at least six hours abstinence from all oral intake and consideration of the need for antacids, H_2-blocking drugs, and careful choice of anaesthetic technique and skilful airway manipulation should all be considered.

The emergency patient

Another group of patients who may have altered gastric physiology are those involved in physical trauma. Gastric emptying is often delayed in these patients due to the stress reaction, pain, and subsequent use of opiates. The central nervous system may be obtunded, leading to a reduced ability to protect the airway. Gastric acid production may also be increased.[41] Regardless of the duration of fasting, these patients must be considered to have full stomachs. Reports of regurgitation of solid and identifiable food over a week post injury have made it clear that the fasting time is an unreliable predictor of gastric emptying. The time interval between the last meal and injury is a more useful determinant of the state of stomach. Similarly, the patient reporting they feel hungry does not indicate that the stomach is empty.[42] As gastric emptying may have ceased at the time of the injury, to insist on normal fasting times and delay surgery does not confer greater safety. Close consultation with surgical colleagues is recommended to optimise the time for both anaesthesia and surgery.

Attempts to empty the stomach in a recently injured patient who needs urgent surgery have been made with the emetic apomorphine and with large-bore nasogastric tubes. Needless to say, neither technique is popular with patients nor can either guarantee an empty stomach. The use of prokinetic agents such as metoclopramide has been advocated by some, and may help.[43]

After a physical injury or medical condition causing shock, the stomach should be assumed to be full. The practitioner may wish to consider the different techniques above to reduce the gastric volume and minimise particulate matter in the stomach, but should general anaesthesia be inevitable, airway protection is essential. Patients who receive a regional anaesthetic are still at risk of aspiration from unexpected complications such as airway compromise due to overzealous sedation or intravascular injection.

A rapid-sequence induction is often employed as a technique to secure and protect the airway rapidly but its use does not guarantee safety nor protect from 'faulty technique. The majority of aspirations occur during intubation despite the use of cricoid pressure. The use of suxamethonium can lead to a rise in intragastric pressure secondary to the fasciculations overcoming the barrier pressure of the lower oesophageal sphincter.[44] Other predisposing factors include an inadequate level of anaesthesia or muscle relaxation and difficult laryngoscopy.[19]

The paediatric patient

Children are at higher risk of aspiration when compared to adults and so must be considered separately. Olsson and colleagues found the incidence of aspiration in children aged 0–9 years to be 8.6 per 10 000 anaesthetics, compared with 2.9 per 10 000 anaesthetics in adults.[45] Indeed, it is believed that regurgitation is normal in the first six months of life, with 30% of children remaining symptomatic until the age of 4 years.[28] Thus 60% of children who aspirated had no preexisting risk factors, but all had problems with airway management. The majority of patients suffered no sequelae.[45]

Various factors combine to increase the risk of gastro–oesophageal reflux in normal children: the relative small size of the stomach, pressure from the abdominal organs, and the ease of gastric inflation from air swallowing or incorrect airway management raise the intragastric pressure, overcoming the lower oesophageal sphincter. The neonate may have transient relaxation of the lower oesophageal sphincter, a less well-developed cough reflex or congenital laryngeal abnormalities.[28] The need to use uncuffed tracheal cuffs in the prepubertal patient reduces the degree of airway protection obtained by intubation. Skilled airway management is therefore paramount in helping prevent gastro–oesophageal reflux and aspiration in these patients.

Despite this, the traditional advice to parents of "nil by mouth" from midnight has now been found to be unnecessary. There is evidence which shows that drinking unlimited clear fluids up to two hours before the predicted time of surgery does not increase and may actually decrease the residual gastric volume and acidity of gastric contents. It has been shown that there is no correlation between the duration of fasting and gastric volume or pH; less than 50% of children had a residual gastric volume of less than 0.4 ml/kg and a pH greater than 2.5 regardless of the fasting time.[32,46,47] Many authors conclude their studies by suggesting that withholding clear fluids for more than two hours preoperatively offers no benefit in terms of minimising volume or acidity of gastric contents.

Breast milk and formulas need to be considered as solids when referring to gastric emptying. Breast milk has a pH of 6.7–7.4 and a fat content that depends on various factors such as maternal diet, time of feed, and interval between feeds.[48] A gastric emptying half-time of 25 minutes for breast milk and 51 minutes for formula milk implies that 95% of the fluid will be

157

emptied within 1.25 or 2.5 hours respectively.[49] Sethi compared the rate of gastric emptying of glucose, low-fat milk, and breast milk by real-time ultrasound.[50] In concordance with prior studies, he showed that a glucose solution was emptied within 1.75 hours and low-fat and breast milk by 2.75 hours. He suggests that low-fat milk in a volume of 10 ml/kg (maximum of 100 ml) can be given up to three hours preoperatively with no added risk. In those children fed breast milk, 13% had residual gastric volumes that put them in the "at-risk" category, leading to the recommendation that breast milk should not be the last feed prior to surgery.[50] Other studies show that despite a large residual gastric volume following a breast feed two hours prior to induction of anaesthesia, no complications of aspiration were noted. It was noted also that the gastric contents had a pH above 7 reflecting the alkaline pH of breast milk.[51] Larger studies need to be performed to fully assess the emptying of breast and low-fat milk from the stomach.

Little work has been performed with regards to altering the duration of the solid fast. This is not surprising in view of the potentially serious complications and the relatively small benefit that shortening the time would bring. One study of children between the ages of one and 14 years compared the residual gastric volume of those given orange squash alone to those given squash and two biscuits.[52] In those fed the biscuits 2–4 hours previously, 40% had food particles in the gastric aspirate compared to 6% who had fasted for six hours, and none in those fasted for longer than six hours.

Recent ASA Practice Guidelines for preoperative fasting recommend that clear fluids may be taken orally up to two hours preoperatively and breast milk may be taken up to four hours before induction of anaesthesia. The fast for formula and solids should exceed eight hours preoperatively.[53] A more liberal approach seems to be taken in the United Kingdom, allowing formula milk to be taken up to 4–6 hours preoperatively.[50]

Pharmacological modification of gastric physiology

In patients with altered gastric physiology, the use of pharmacological adjuvants to enhance gastric emptying, raise lower oesophageal sphincter tone and increase the gastric pH should be considered. The use of multiple agents confers no additional benefit.[19,54] Many patients with gastric symptomatology present for surgery established on some of the medications considered below. These should be continued in the perioperative period. See also Chapter 9.

Promoting gastric emptying

Prokinetic agents
Prokinetic agents such as the dopamine antagonist metoclopramide enhance the rate of gastric emptying, increase the lower oesophageal sphincter tone and are antiemetic. Metodopramide has no effect on gastric secretion or

pH.[55] It is often used in obstetric anaesthesia, for patients with a hiatus hernia and for those patients in whom there is inadequate time for gastric emptying due to the need for urgent surgery. The cholinergic agonist cisapride also promotes gastric emptying (see p. 173 for the most recent information concerning cisa pride).

Anticholinergic drugs

Anticholinergic drugs such as atropine, hyoscine, and glycopyrrolate act on the gastric cholinergic muscarinic receptors to reduce gastric secretion and ultimately volume. This effect is best demonstrated after large intravenous doses, limiting their clinical usefulness. Further disadvantages due to an inhibition of gastric motility and relaxation of the lower oesophageal sphincter make them unsuitable for acid aspiration prophylaxis.[24]

Raising gastric pH

Simple antacids

Antacids are alkaline liquids which raise the gastric pH by direct neutralisation of acid. Their effectiveness is limited by the degree of mixing that occurs after ingestion, the volume and pH of acid to be neutralised, the increased gastric volume subsequent to and the timing of their administration. Particulate antacids such as magnesium trisilicate should be avoided as aspiration of particulate matter may cause acute pulmonary obstruction and a chronic granulomatous inflammatory response.[56] Antacid prophylaxis against pulmonary aspiration has become popular and is routinely administered prior to general and regional anaesthesia in obstetric practice.

Histamine H₂-receptor antagonists

Histamine receptor antagonists are competitive inhibitors of the H_2 receptor on the gastric parietal cell and act to reduce gastric acid secretion. Ranitidine is the preferred drug of this class, having fewer side effects and a longer duration of action than cimetidine.

Proton pump inhibitors

Omeprazole, a proton pump inhibitor, has been shown to be as effective as ranitidine when used in equipotent doses prior to surgery.[57] By these actions, these two classes of drugs also lower gastric volume.

Guidelines

The most recent published guidelines for the selection of preoperative fasting regimens and use of pharmacological agents to reduce the risk of pulmonary aspiration have come from the USA. The ASA established a task force to review and analyse the relevant published research on the subject and formulate evidence-based recommendations. International opinions were canvassed prior to a consensus view being published. These guidelines only refer to the healthy patient undergoing elective surgery and patients who are not in this category require individual preparations as discussed earlier. Box 8.2 summarises the recommendations with respect to preoperative evaluation and preparation of the normal patient.[53]

The guidelines state that insufficient studies of the relationship between reduced gastric acid secretion and the frequency of aspiration in humans have been performed. There is also insufficient evidence to evaluate whether pharmacological manipulation to reduce gastric acid secretion, lower gastric volume or raise gastric pH is actually associated with decreased morbidity or mortality in those who have aspirated gastric contents. The ASA recommends that there should be no routine use of pharmacological agents to alter gastric contents and pH unless indicated by the presence of significant risk factors and that anticholinergics are not recommended in any circumstances.[53]

Different countries have published alternative guidelines which were reviewed in 1996.[58] To contrast with the American guidelines, only the differences will be stated (Box 8.3).

Box 8.2 Guidelines for the selection of preoperative fasting regimens for healthy patients undergoing elective surgery[53]

Preoperative assessment
- A full history, physical examination and review of the medical records looking for evidence of risk factors for gastro–oesophageal reflux and aspiration should be performed
- At this time patients should be informed of their fasting times in a written and verbal form

Fasting times for clear fluids
- Water, pulpless fruit juices, black tea and coffee may be taken until two hours preoperatively
- The volume of fluid taken appears to be less important than the actual type of fluid

Fasting times for breast milk
- A fasting time of four hours is recommended

Fasting times for infant formula
- A fasting time of six hours is recommended

Fasting times for solids and non-human milk
- A fasting time of six hours is recommended for a light meal or non-human milk
- Fried, fatty foods or meat may require a longer fasting time
- The amount of food ingested also needs to be taken into consideration

---

Box 8.3 National variations in preoperative fasting regimens for healthy patients undergoing elective surgery[54]

Canada
- No solid food on the day of surgery
- Unrestricted clear fluids until three hours prior to surgery

United Kingdom
- No actual formal guidelines have been printed but it appears to be similar to the American report

Denmark
- Clear fluids allowed up to four hours prior to anaesthesia

Norway
- 250 ml of tea, coffee, lemonade or water up to two hours before anaesthesia
- A "light meal" can be taken four hours before

Sweden
- No solid food from midnight on the day of surgery
- Clear soup or yoghurt allowed up to four hours prior to surgery
- Clear fluids allowed 2–3 hours prior to surgery

Conclusion

Over the past decade the instructions regarding preoperative fasting have changed by allowing patients to drink clear fluids much closer to the time of induction of anaesthesia. This is not because it has been shown to be safer with regards to the risks of aspiration and pulmonary damage, but because there is no added benefit of the prolonged fast for fluids. Patients' well-being has also been shown to be improved. Solid food continues to be withheld for longer periods of time, but with more accurate methods of measuring gastric emptying rates, these guidelines may be changed in the future.

The effects of these new guidelines may be difficult to assess. The low incidence of pulmonary pathology following aspiration and the subjective nature of the benefits make outcome studies difficult to perform. The increase in day stay surgery and staggered admissions to hospital will possibly lead to reluctance to change and because traditional fasting times have almost become anaesthetic "folklore", it may take time for these guidelines to become accepted.

1   Snow J. *On the inhalation of the vapour of ether in surgical operations.* London: Churchill, 1847: 43–4.
2   Snow J. *On chloroform and other anaesthesia.* London: Churchill, 1858: 74–5.
3   Lister J. On anaesthetics, Part 3. In: *Holmes' system of surgery,* vol 3, 3rd edn. London 1883 (reprinted in *The collected papers of Joseph Lister.* Birmingham: Classics of Medicine Library, 1979: 171–2).

4   Simpson JY. Remarks on the alleged case of death from the action of chloroform. *Lancet* 1848; **1**: 175.

5   Mendelson CL. The aspiration of stomach contents into the lungs during obstetric anaesthesia. *Am J Obstet Gynecol* 1946; **53**: 191–205.

6   Teabut JR. Aspiration of gastric contents: an experimental study. *Am J Pathol* 1952; **28**: 51–62.

7   Beaumont W. *Gastric juice and the physiology of digestion.* Pittsburgh: Allen, 1833: 277, 159–60.

8   Minami H, McCallum R. The physiology and pathology of gastric emptying in humans. *Gastroenterology* 1984; **86**: 1592–806.

9   Petring OU, Blake DW. Gastric emptying in adults: an overview related to anaesthesia. *Anaesth Intens Care* 1993; **21**: 774–81.

10 Stoelting RK, ed. *Pharmacology and physiology in anesthetic practice*, 2nd edn. Philadelphia: Lippincott, 1991: 782–94.

11 Tryba M, Mlasowsky B, Huchzermeyer H. Does a stomach tube enhance regurgitation during general anaesthesia? *Anaesthetist* 1983; **32**: 407–9.

12 Hardy JF, Lepagr Y, Bonville-Chouinard N. Occurrence of gastrooesophageal reflux on induction of anaesthesia does not correlate with the volume of gastric contents. *Can J Anaesth* 1990; **37**: 502–8.

13 Bosomworth PP, Hamelberg W. The etiologic and therapeutic aspects of aspiration pneumonitis: experimental study. *Surg Forum* 1962; **13**: 158–9.

14 Roberts RB, Shirley MA. Reducing the risk of acid aspiration syndrome during cesarian section. *Anesth Analg* 1974; **53**: 859–68.

15 Awe WB, Fletcher WS, Jacob SW. Pathophysiology of aspiration pneumonitis. *Surgery* 1966; **60**: 232–9.

16 Exarhos ND, Logan WD Jr, Abbot OA *et al.* The importance of pH and volume in tracheobronchial aspiration. *Dis Chest* 1965; **47**: 167–9.

17 Raidoo DM, Rocke JG, Brock-Utne JG *et al.* Critical volume for pulmonary acid aspiration reappraisal in a primate model. *Br J Anaesth* 1990; **65**: 248–50.

18 Olsson GL, Hallen B, Hambraeus-Jonzon K. Aspiration during anaesthesia: a computer-aided study of 185,358 anaesthetics. *Acta Anaesthesiol Scand* 1986; **30**: 84–92.

19 Warner MA, Warner ME, Weber JG. Clinical significance of pulmonary aspiration during the perioperative period. *Anesthesiology* 1993; **78**: 56–62.

20 Miller M, Wishart HY, Nimmo WS. Gastric contents at induction of anaesthesia. Is a 4 hour fast necessary? *Br J Anaesth* 1983; **55**: 1185–7.

21 Maltby JR, Lewis P, Martin A *et al.* Gastric fluid volume and pH in elective patients following unrestricted oral fluid intake until three hours before surgery. *Can J Anaesth* 1991; **38**: 425–9.

22 Phillips S, Hutchinson S, Davidson T. Preoperative drinking does not affect gastric contents. *Br J Anaesth* 1993; **70**: 6–9.

23 Agarwal A, Chari P, Singh H. Fluid deprivation before operation. *Anaesthesia* 1989; **44**: 632–4.

24 Kallar S, Everett L. Potential risks and preventative measures for pulmonary aspiration: new concepts in preoperative fasting guidelines. *Anesth Analg* 1993; **77**: 171–82.

25 Goodwin APL, Rowe WL, Ogg TW *et al.* Oral fluids prior to day surgery. *Anaesthesia* 1991; **46**: 1066–8.

26 Miller DC. Why are children starved? *Br J Anaesth* 1990; **64**: 409–10.

27 Salem MR, Wong AY, Collins VJ. The paediatric patient with a full stomach. *Anesthesiology* 1973; **39**: 435–9.

28 Phillips S, Daboran AK, Hatch DJ. Preoperative fasting for paediatric anaesthesia. *Br J Anaesth* 1994; **73**: 529–36.

29 Redfern N, Addison GM, Meakin G. Blood glucose in anaesthetised children. *Anaesthesia* 1986; **42**: 272–5.

30 Thomas DKM. Hypoglycaemia in children before operation: its incidence and prevention. *Br J Anaesth* 1974; **46**: 66–8.

31 Payne K, Ireland P. Plasma glucose in the peri-operative period in children. *Anaesthesia* 1984; **39**: 868–72.

32 Schreiner MS, Triebwasser A, Keon TP. Ingestion of liquids compared with preoperative fasting in pediatric outpatients. *Anesthesiology* 1990; **72**: 593–7.

162

33 Gilbert SS, Easy WR, Fitch WW. The effect of oral fluids on morbidity following anaesthesia for minor surgery. *Anaesthesia* 1995; **50**: 79–81.

34 Cobley M, Dunne JA, Sanders LD. Stressful pre-operative preparation procedures. *Anaesthesia* 1991; **46**: 1019–22.

35 Read MS, Vaughan RS. Allowing preoperative patients to drink: effects on patients' safety and comfort of unlimited oral water until two hours before anaesthesia. *Acta Anaesthesiol Scand* 1991; **35**: 591–5.

36 Gibbs CP, Modell JH. Pulmonary aspiration of gastric contents. In: Miller RD, ed. *Anesthesia*, 4th edn. New York: Churchill Livingstone, 1994: 1437–64.

37 Beischer NA, Mackay EV, eds. *The management of normal labour: analgesia and anaesthesia*, 2nd edn. Sydney: Saunders, 1991: 350–63.

38 Scrutton MJL, Metcalfe GA, Seed PT *et al.* Eating in labour. *Anaesthesia* 1999; **54**: 329–34.

39 Harter RL, Kelly WB, Kramer MG *et al.* A comparison of the volume and pH of gastric contents of obese and lean surgical patients. *Anesth Analg* 1998; **86**: 147–52.

40 Roizen MF. Anaesthetic implications and concurrent disease. In: Miller RD, ed. *Anesthesia*, 4th edn. New York: Churchill Livingstone, 1994: 903–1014.

41 Schurizer BA, Rybro L, Boggild-Madsen NB *et al.* Gastric volume and pH in children for emergency surgery. *Acta Anaesthesiol Scand* 1986; **30**: 404–8.

42 Bricker SR, McLuckie A, Nightingale A. Gastric aspirates after trauma in children. *Anaesthesia* 1989; **44**: 721–4.

43 Stene JK, Grande CM. Anesthesia for trauma. In: Miller RD, ed. *Anesthesia*, 4th edn. New York: Churchill Livingstone, 1994: 2157–73.

44 Muravchick S, Burkett L, Gold MI. Succinylcholine-induced fasciculations and intragastric pressure during induction of anaesthesia. *Anesthesiology* 1982; **55**: 180–3.

45 Tiret L, Nivoche Y, Hatton F *et al.* Complications related to anaesthesia in infants and children. A prospective study of 40240 anaesthetics. *Br J Anaesth* 1988; **62**: 263–9.

46 Ingebo K, Rayborn N, Hecht R *et al.* Sedation in children: adequacy of two hour fasting. *J Pediatr* 1997; **131**: 155–8.

47 Splinter WM, Schaeffer JC. Unlimited clear fluid ingestion two hours before surgery does not affect volume or pH of stomach contents. *Anaesth Intens Care* 1990; **18**: 522–6.

48 Litman RS, Wu CL, Quinlivan K. Gastric volume and pH in infants fed clear liquids and breast milk prior to surgery. *Anesth Analg* 1994; **79**: 482–5.

49 Cavell B. Gastric emptying in infants fed human milk or infant formula. *Acta Paediatr Scand* 1981; **70**: 639–41.

50 Sethi AK, Chatterji C, Bhargava SK *et al.* Safe pre-operative fasting times after milk or clear fluid in children. A preliminary study using real time ultrasound. *Anaesthesia* 1998; **54**: 51–85.

51 van der Walt JH, Foate JA, Murrell D *et al.* A study of preoperative fasting in infants aged less than three months. *Anaesth Intens Care* 1990; **18**: 527–31.

52 Meakin G, Dingwall AE, Addison GM. Effects of fasting and oral premedication on the pH and volume of gastric aspirate in children. *Br J Anaesth* 1987; **59**: 678–82.

53 American Society of Anesthesiologists. Practice guidelines for preoperative fasting and the use of pharmacologic agents to reduce the risk of pulmonary aspiration: application to healthy patients undergoing elective procedures. *Anesthesiology* 1999; **90**: 896–905.

54 Maltby JR, Warnell I, Sutherland LR *et al.* Gastric fluid volume and pH in elective surgical patients: triple therapy is not superior to ranitidine alone. *Can J Anaesth* 1990; **37**: 650–5.

55 Reynolds JC, Putnam PE. Prokinetic agents. *Gastroenterol Clin North Am* 1992; **21**: 567–96.

56 McCammon RL. Prophylaxis for aspiration pneumonitis. In: *ASA annual refresher course lectures*. Hagersdown: American Society of Anesthesiologists, 1986: 224.

57 Atanassof PG, Alon E, Pasch T. Effects of single dose intravenous omeprazole and ranitidine on gastric pH during general anaesthesia. *Anesth Analg* 1992; **73**: 95–8.

58 Eriksson LI, Sandin R. Fasting guidelines in different countries. *Acta Anaesthesiol Scand* 1996; **40**: 971–4.

9: Premedication

CARL GWINNUTT, ANTHONY McCLUSKEY

The term "premedication" dates from the 1920s[1] and was originally an abbreviation of "preliminary medication", although it is synonymous with preanaesthetic and preoperative medication. It generally refers to drugs administered to patients before induction of anaesthesia, usually but not exclusively prescribed by anaesthetists. Preoperative medication can be considered to have long predated general anaesthesia as alcohol, opium, and mandrake (a source of hyoscine and other alkaloids) were commonly given to produce a degree of stupefaction and analgesia in those poor unfortunates requiring surgery.

Although the technique of premedication has been used widely since the first successful demonstration of general anaesthesia in 1846,[2] the principal aims and objectives have altered over the years in conjunction with changes in the practice of general anaesthesia itself. In the earlier years, premedicant drugs were used to facilitate smooth induction of anaesthesia, to reduce the amount of inhalational agent required to produce surgical anaesthesia and to decrease the frequency of side effects associated with the use of chloroform and ether. In 1869, the French physiologist Claude Bernard described how morphine given preoperatively to dogs resulted in smoother, more rapid induction of anaesthesia using a smaller dose of chloroform, a practice rapidly adopted by many anaesthetists. However, it was by no means universal, in part due to the associated problem of respiratory depression. The use of atropine as a premedicant became popular at the turn of the century following the discovery that it opposed the cardioinhibitory vagal effects of deep chloroform anaesthesia. Although atropine probably prevented a number of chloroform-related deaths in this way, the majority of fatalities were due in fact to ventricular fibrillation during induction of anaesthesia with chloroform.

In the early 20th century, chloroform was gradually superseded by ether, a safer agent causing less cardiovascular depression and reduced tendency to provoke dysrhythmias. An inconvenient side effect of ether inhalation was stimulation of salivary and bronchial secretions and so atropine premedication remained popular because of its anticholinergic antisialogogue action. Hyoscine (scopolamine) was also used for the same reason and had the additional advantages of possessing antiemetic, sedative, and amnesic properties. It remained popular in the UK until relatively recently and was often prescribed in combination with Omnopon (papaveretum, a mixture of opium alkaloids) and colloquially refered to as "Om & Scop". This popularity was probably due at least in part to the popularity of thiopentone, nitrous oxide, oxygen, and muscle relaxant anaesthesia (the Liverpool technique) which omitted an anaesthetic vapour and was associated with a risk of intraoperative awareness in unpremedicated patients.

However, this practice is now much less popular as modern drugs, in particular potent, well-tolerated, inhalational and intravenous agents, do not rely upon premedication to facilitate induction or maintenance of anaesthesia. It has also been recognised that one of the main aims of premedication, namely the reduction of patient anxiety, is not reliably achieved using opioids. With the discovery of the benzodiazepines in the 1960s, anaesthetists now possessed reliable anxiolytic drugs, which could be administered orally, thus avoiding the need for painful intramuscular injections. Today, oral benzodiazepines remain the most commonly prescribed premedicant drugs.[3] However, anaesthetists are now questioning the need for pharmacological premedication, certainly as a routine aspect of modern anaesthetic practice.[4]

In the USA, injection of intravenous benzodiazepines or opioids just prior to anaesthesia is sometimes also considered to be premedication. However, we would prefer to use the term "co-induction of anaesthesia" for this technique.

Aims of premedication

The primary aims of premedication for most surgical procedures are summarised in Box 9.1, "The six As of premedication".[5] A premedicant drug or combination of drugs may possess one or more of these properties. It is not difficult to envisage clinical scenarios where all six attributes would be desirable. In addition to these primary aims of premedication, there are a number of special situations where other considerations apply, usually as a result of the need to ensure continuation of a patient's medical treatment or prophylaxis against certain perioperative events.

Box 9.1 The six As of premedication

- Anxiolysis
- Amnesia
- Analgesia
- Antiemesis
- Antacid
- Antiautonomic

Anxiolysis

A whole spectrum of anxiety may be experienced by patients awaiting surgery. Its frequency and intensity will depend on how it is defined (psychological calmness, sedation, sympathoadrenal activity), measured (visual analogue scale (VAS) scores, verbal response scale (VRS) scores, psychological questionnaires, stress hormone levels, physical signs of anxiety) and who measures it (patient, anaesthetist, psychologist).[6] Although it is important to alleviate preoperative anxiety on humanitarian grounds, as Guedel first noted in 1937, anxious patients appear to "resist" induction of anaesthesia[7] and are more likely to experience a "stormy" induction.[8] This phenomenon is probably due to stimulation of the reticular activating system by circulating catecholamines, along with a tachycardia, hypertension, and even dysrhythmias or myocardial ischaemia in susceptible patients. There is also some evidence that anxious patients require more postoperative analgesia and recover less quickly from the effects of anaesthesia and surgery.[9,10]

In the context of premedication, it is common to consider only the preoperative anxiety experienced by patients in the final run-up to surgery. However, patients' anxiety may be raised for several days before and be sustained for several days after surgery.[11] Only in a minority of patients does anxiety appear to peak on the day of surgery itself.[12] Although patients are often anxious about either anaesthesia or surgery, they sometimes have other worries such as work, family and intrusion into their personal privacy by acts such as removal of dentures.

Therefore, pharmacological premedication, one or two hours before surgery, cannot be a panacea for preoperative anxiety. It is at least as important that those involved in the perioperative care of patients should attempt to identify and manage sources of anxiety and stress appropriately, and at an early stage. An adequate explanation and reassurance at the initial consultation with the surgeon is beneficial and the provision of booklets and audio-visual aids has been shown to reduce preoperative anxiety levels significantly.[9,10] Despite this, one of the principal aims of the anaesthetist's preoperative visit is to allay specific patient fears such as "Will I be asleep?" and "Will I wake up?". Conducted sympathetically, the preoperative visit is often more effective than pharmacological anxiolysis.[13,14] Nevertheless, many patients will still benefit from anxiolytic premedication. If the anaesthetist visits the patient on the day before surgery, it may be appropriate to prescribe a long-acting drug with sedative and anxiolytic properties such as diazepam or lorazepam for that evening and again if necessary the following morning.

Although the benzodiazepines are the most commonly prescribed premedicants, other drugs are sometimes used to provide preoperative anxiolysis and sedation. Historically, barbiturates were used but have now been superseded because of the profound respiratory and cardiovascular depression associated with their use. Neuroleptics produce sedation and anxiolysis and are also effective antiemetics. However, the side effects of extrapyramidal symptoms, oculogyric crises and anticholinergic actions (for example, blurred vision and dry mouth, hypotension, and unpleasant psychological sequelae) limit their use. Low-dose droperidol is sometimes given with a benzodiazepine as the combination seems to provide reliable anxiolysis, sedation, and effective antiemesis with an acceptably low incidence of adverse side effects. β-blockers may be useful in selective patients in whom palpitations as a result of anxiety-induced tachycardia and hypertension are a particular problem. Opioids should not be used for preoperative anxiolysis. Although they do cause sedation, contrary to popular belief they are not usually euphoric and do not relieve anxiety in this context. Indeed, dysphoria is produced in 80% of normal control subjects.[15] Furthermore, there are the unwanted side effects of nausea and vomiting, delayed gastric emptying, itching, and respiratory depression.

Despite the recognition that preoperative anxiety is one of the main concerns of both patients and their anaesthetists, on the whole it is a subjective experience and therefore presents a problem in both definition and measurement. Numerous pitfalls in the design and methodology of previous studies of anxiolytic premedication mean that it is difficult to compare the relative merits of different premedicants.[6,16]

Benzodiazepines
Benzodiazepines were introduced in 1960 with the synthesis of chlordiazepoxide (Librium) and although a large family of drugs, only three or four are commonly used for preoperative anxiolysis in the UK. The benzodiazepines act at specific receptors within the brain which are associated with, although distinct from, inhibitory gamma-aminobutyric acid (GABA) receptors. They have a variety of actions: anxiolysis, sedation, anterograde amnesia, anticonvulsant, and muscle relaxation (central in origin). The degree of each of these actions varies between each drug. They are neither emetic nor antiemetic. Flumazenil, a specific benzodiazepine receptor antagonist, is available in cases of overdosage. Although oral benzodiazepines are generally not considered to cause significant cardiovascular or respiratory depression at recommended doses, caution must be exercised in the elderly, in patients with cardiac disease, a reduced level of consciousness as a result of raised intracranial pressure and when given concurrently with opioids.

Diazepam. Diazepam has been studied extensively and is effective in relieving preoperative anxiety and producing sedation when given at a dose of 5–20 mg.[17–23] Its amnesic potential is less than that of midazolam and lorazepam. The effects of diazepam after oral administration are reliable although it must be given at least one hour prior to anaesthesia. The simultaneous administration of metoclopramide (Maxolon) increases both the peak plasma concentration of diazepam and the speed with which it is achieved by increasing gastric emptying. Conversely, concurrently administered opioids and atropine have the opposite effect. Diazepam is available for parenteral use as a solution in propylene glycol and as a lipid emulsion (Diazemuls). The former is an irritant, causing pain on intramuscular injection and unpredictable absorption and may cause thrombophlebitis when given intravenously. The elimination half-life of diazepam is greater than 24 hours and that of desmethyldiazepam, the principal active metabolite, is even longer. The elimination half-life of diazepam rises with age, reaching approximately 90 hours in octogenarians. Diazepam may therefore produce unnecessary and prolonged sedation, which may be advantageous when the timing of surgery is unpredictable but contraindicated in day surgery.

Lorazepam. Lorazepam is approximately four times as potent as diazepam and is an effective preoperative anxiolytic at an oral dose of 1–4 mg.[23-27] It may also be given by intramuscular injection. As the latency of action is longer than that of diazepam, due in part to its slow penetration of the CSF,[28] lorazepam should be given at least 90 minutes prior to anaesthesia. The duration of useful anxiolysis and sedation is similarly long and may last all day so that there is flexibility in the timing of administration relative to surgery. The elimination half-life of lorazepam is approximately 15 hours and there are no active metabolites. The amnesic effect is more marked than that of diazepam and following premedication, patients will often have little or no recollection of events occurring on the day of surgery. Whilst profound amnesia may occasionally be a desirable goal for either anaesthetist or patient, it could clearly be a significant problem, for example in the context of day surgery.

Temazepam. Temazepam is an active metabolite of diazepam and is used for premedication at a dose of 10–40 mg orally.[29-34] It is more rapidly absorbed from the gastrointestinal tract than either diazepam or lorazepam and peak levels are usually achieved within 30–60 minutes. Although the plasma half-life is approximately 12 hours, the clinically useful duration of action is certainly less than this and necessitates relatively accurate timing in relation to the start of surgery. Consequently, if for any reason surgery is delayed, it is not uncommon for the patient to declare that he has had a relaxing sleep but that the premedication has now "worn off". However, the short duration of action is an asset in day surgery where it has been used successfully at a dose of 10–20 mg with minimal hangover or delay in discharge. Amnesia is not a prominent feature of its use.

Midazolam. Midazolam is a water-soluble, rapid-onset, short-acting benzo-diazepine with an elimination half-life of only 2–3 hours, with no active metabolites. The oral bioavailabilty of midazolam is only approximately 30–50% due to extensive first-pass hepatic metabolism, but its efficacy as a premedicant has been demonstrated in a number of studies.[29,31,32] It is usually given orally at a dose of 7.5–15 mg, 30–60 minutes preoperatively and has a short duration of action, with an amnesic effect greater than that of diazepam. Sublingual midazolam may be more effective than the oral route.[35] Midazolam is particularly useful in day surgery when the interval between premedication and surgery may be short and where rapid recovery from the residual effects of anaesthesia is necessary. Oral midazolam (0.5 mg/kg) is also widely used in paediatric anaesthesia where the amnesia induced may be advantageous in reducing the incidence of psychological sequaelae following anaesthesia and surgery.[36,37] Midazolam has also been administered intranasally (0.2–0.3 mg/kg) to children, producing sedation and anxiolysis within 10–15 minutes.

Unfortunately, midazolam is not licensed for oral use in several countries including the UK, nor is it available in tablet form. It is therefore usually given as the intravenous preparation mixed with a small volume of syrup to make it more palatable. Midazolam tablets are available elsewhere in Europe as Dormicum 7.5 mg and 15 mg. In the USA, midazolam is the most commonly used benzodiazepine premedicant, although due to differences in practice, it is usually given by intramuscular or intravenous injection shortly before induction of anaesthesia.

Amnesia

Although amnesia is included as one of the basic aims of premedication, it is open to debate as to whether it should be considered more appropriately as a side effect of some premedicant drugs. Certainly, there are a group of patients who express a desire not to remember any perioperative events, although these are probably a small minority.[38] Amnesia is useful if it clouds memories of potentially unpleasant preoperative procedures (for example, insertion of invasive haemodynamic monitoring lines, institution of regional blockade). However, its attainment is not an excuse for awareness under light general anaesthesia or inadequate or ineffective analgesia in the imme-diate postoperative period. Perioperative amnesia may be more important in paediatric anaesthesia as children have been shown to exhibit disturbed psychological behaviour following hospital admission for surgery.[36,39] Amnesia is best avoided in day surgery patients as they may forget important postoperative instructions and return to "normal" activities sooner than advised. Premedicant drugs with significant amnesic effects include lorazepam and midazolam and the anticholinergic agent hyoscine. The amnesia is characteristically anterograde.

Analgesia

Opioids were the first premedicant drugs but have now been replaced with more effective and safer anxiolytic drugs. Their use should be limited to patients in pain prior to surgery when they should be given parenterally because of delayed absorption following oral administration, and in combination with an antiemetic. As opioids are not very effective anxiolytics, it is possible to achieve a well-sedated but still terrified patient if they are given alone. The side effect profile of opioids is well known. Potentially dangerous respiratory and cardiovascular depression may occur when opioids are given in combination with a benzodiazepine. Although the dose range of morphine is usually quoted as 0.1–0.2 mg/kg, it is not really possible to recommend a dosage schedule for opioid drugs as the dose–response relationship is subject to so many interindividual variations. Rather, the drug should be carefully titrated against the patient's pain.

In recent years there has been a revival in the subject of analgesic premedication following the description of the concept of preemptive analgesia. Currently, evidence as to whether opioid and non-steroidal analgesics are more effective when given preoperatively is conflicting.[40]

Antiemesis

Postoperative nausea and vomiting (PONV) are common and frequently distressing sequelae of anaesthesia, surgery, and opioid analgesia. More common in women than men and in younger patients, the aetiology is multifactorial.[41] Not surprisingly, therefore, antiemetics are often used as premedicants in order to try and prevent PONV. Unfortunately, none of the currently available antiemetic drugs can be relied upon either to prevent or treat established PONV. It is also difficult to make accurate comparisons between different treatment regimes due to differences in methodology between trials, such as the type of surgery and anaesthesia, the patient population and the definition and measurement of PONV itself (Box 9.2).[16]

Furthermore, the rationale for premedicating patients with oral antiemetics is somewhat open to question as it is probably more logical to prevent PONV by giving such drugs intravenously following induction of anaesthesia.

Box 9.2 Antiemetic drugs used as premedicants

- Dopamine antagonists – metoclopramide, prochlorperazine
- Antihistamines – promethazine, trimeprazine
- Neuroleptic agents – droperidol
- 5-HT$_3$ antagonists – ondansetron, granisetron
- Anticholinergic agents – hyoscine, atropine

Specific antiemetic drugs

Metoclopramide. Metoclopramide is a dopamine antagonist with several beneficial actions. As well as being an antiemetic, it increases the barrier pressure of the lower oesophageal sphincter and promotes gastric emptying.[42,43] It is a logical choice when delayed gastric emptying is suspected. Although metoclopramide is an effective antiemetic, there is somewhat limited evidence of the efficacy of oral metoclopramide premedication in reducing the incidence of PONV.[44,45] Interestingly, despite being widely used, it is not licensed for use in PONV!

Droperidol. Droperidol is a butyrophenone, a group of drugs which are used in the treatment of schizophrenia and other psychoses. They generally tranquillise without causing sedation, although they do potentiate the sedative effects of concurrently administered benzodiazepines. Troublesome side effects include extrapyramidal symptoms (acute dystonic reactions, akathisia, oculogyric crises), hypotension, hypothermia, unpleasant psychological reactions of inner restlessness and the potential to trigger the malignant neuroleptic syndrome.

The efficacy of droperidol as an effective antiemetic, administered either as an oral premedicant (2.5–5 mg) or intravenously during induction of anaesthesia (0.5–2.5 mg), has been shown in a number of studies.[46–48] Some comparative studies have demonstrated that droperidol may even be as effective as the newer 5-HT$_3$ antagonists in preventing PONV.[49–51] Unfortunately, its side effect profile is unfavourable and many anaesthetists avoid the use of droperidol, although when used in the low doses suggested above it is usually well tolerated.

Ondansetron. Numerous recent studies have described the efficacy of ondansetron and other 5-HT$_3$ antagonists in treating PONV.[52–58] However, most of these have focused on the intravenous route during anaesthesia rather than on oral premedication. A recent large meta analysis of over 12 000 patients given prophylactic ondansetron intravenously concluded that for every six patients treated with intravenous ondansetron 4 mg (the optimal dose), one patient will not vomit as a result of the treatment, two patients will vomit despite the treatment and the remaining three patients would not have vomited anyway.[59] The most effective oral dose of ondansetron is 16 mg administered one hour prior to surgery.[57] The combination of intravenous granisetron 40 μg/kg and droperidol 1.25 mg immediately before induction of anaesthesia produced a remarkable 96% response rate in one study.[55] Ondansetron and related drugs are well tolerated with only headache reported as a significant side effect. The major drawback at present to the routine use of this group of drugs is their relative expense.

Hyoscine. Hyoscine is an effective antiemetic, particularly in preventing motion sickness. However, unacceptable anticholinergic side effects (dry mouth, blurred vision, central anticholinergic syndrome) limit its use when given orally or parenterally. Hyoscine is available as a transdermal patch, which produces very low plasma levels. However, the evidence that it is an effective antiemetic premedicant is conflicting.[60-64]

Antacid

It is important to recognise that in some patients, the stomach may not be empty even though they have been kept "nil by mouth" for an appropriate length of time. Such patients are at risk of acid aspiration (Mendelson's Syndrome) during induction of anaesthesia, before the trachea has been intubated with a cuffed tube (Box 9.3). Both the volume and acidity of gastric secretions aspirated are important determinants of the severity of the subsequent lung injury and several premedicant drugs are useful in either reducing the volume, increasing pH or both (Box 9.4). See also Chapter 8.

Box 9.3 Patients at increased risk of acid aspiration syndrome (volume of gastric contents greater than 0.4 ml/kg, pH less than 2.5)

Delayed gastric emptying or insufficient time for emptying
- Emergency surgery
- Pregnancy
- Pain
- Anxiety
- After opioid or anticholinergic administration
- Systemic illness
- Bowel obstruction

Increased risk of regurgitation
- Obesity
- Pregnancy
- Hiatus hernia
- Oesophageal motility disorders or stricture
- Pharyngeal pouch

Box 9.4 Drugs used to decrease the volume and acidity of gastric secretions

---

- H$_2$-receptor antagonists – cimetidine, ranitidine, famotidine
- Proton pump inhibitors – omeprazole, lansoprazole
- Gastrokinetic agents – metoclopramide, cisapride
- Simple antacids – sodium citrate

Histamine (H₂) receptor antagonists

Histamine (H₂) receptor antagonists

This group of drugs directly inhibit the secretion of gastric acid. Cimetidine, ranitidine and more recently famotidine have been shown to be effective as oral premedicants.[65-71] Unfortunately, cimetidine inhibits the cytochrome P-450 microsomal enzyme system of the liver and may therefore decrease the metabolism and augment the effect of concomitantly administered drugs (for example, diazepam, midazolam, propranolol, warfarin, theophyllines, phenytoin, carbamazepine, bupivacaine). Cimetidine may also cause mental confusion in the elderly.

The most commonly prescribed prophylaxis for aspiration pneumonia in the UK is probably ranitidine, which has been tried and tested for over 20 years. It has minimal adverse side effects or drug interactions and is cheaper than the proton pump inhibitors (see below). Patients at risk of regurgitation and aspiration may be given a dose of 150 mg orally the night before surgery and again the next morning approximately two hours before the time of scheduled surgery. Patients on afternoon operating lists should have their first dose on waking and the second two hours before the time of scheduled surgery.

Proton pump inhibitors

Omeprazole and related drugs inhibit the gastric parietal cellular enzyme hydrogen-potassium-adenosine triphosphatase (the proton pump) which produces hydrochloric acid. They are used extensively in the management of peptic ulcer disease. Like cimetidine, omeprazole also inhibits cytochrome P-450 and must therefore be used with caution with other drugs that are similarly metabolised. There are relatively few data from well-conducted controlled trials comparing H₂-receptor antagonists and proton pump inhibitors in the context of anaesthetic premedication and that which is available is conflicting. Preoperative omeprazole has been shown to be either more,[72] less[69,73] or equally effective[74,75] as an H₂ antagonist in reducing resting gastric volumes and raising pH.

Gastrokinetic agents

Metoclopramide is a dopamine antagonist that promotes gastric emptying and reduces the risk of oesophageal regurgitation by tightening the lower oesophageal sphincter. It is often administered in combination with ranitidine. Although cisapride is effective at reducing fasting gastric volume[76] and reversing the delay in gastric emptying due to morphine,[77] it has recently been withdrawn by the manufacturers as a result of an unacceptably high incidence of cardiac arrhythmias.*

---

* On 28th July 2000, the Medicines Control Agency of the UK Department of Health withdrew the license for cisapride. The license for cisapride is under review in many European countries.

Simple antacids

Sodium citrate (0.3 M, 3 ml), is used almost universally in the UK, in conjunction with an H_2 antagonist, in parturients scheduled for elective or emergency caesarean section. The combination of preoperative oral sodium citrate and ranitidine has been shown to be more effective than ranitidine alone.[78] The antacid is given immediately before the start of anaesthesia. The patient must be warned of its foul taste. Once ingested, many anaesthetists insist on rotating the patient to ensure as far as possible that thorough mixing of the entire residual gastric contents results. Sodium citrate is non-particulate and is therefore more suitable than particulate antacids such as magnesium trisilicate, which may provoke an inflammatory reaction within the lungs if aspirated.

Antiautonomic effects

Anticholinergic effects

Atropine and hyoscine have been used as premedicants from the early days of anaesthesia, either to antagonise the vagotonic effect of chloroform or as an antisialogogue when using ether. As recently as 20 years ago approximately 20% of practising UK anaesthetists were still using them routinely[79] but they are now considered largely unnecessary with modern anaesthetic drugs, apart from a few special circumstances (Box 9.5).

For patients, the accompanying dry mouth and sore throat can be most unpleasant and thickening of bronchial secretions makes their expectoration more difficult and may lead to postoperative atelectasis and pneumonia. Other unwanted side effects of anticholinergic premedication include blurred vision, urinary retention, relaxation of the lower oesophageal sphincter, delayed gastric emptying, reduced gastrointestinal motility, tachycardia, dysrhythmias, and inhibition of sweating.

Atropine and hyoscine are tertiary amines and thus readily cross the blood–brain barrier. Atropine has excitatory effects on the CNS whereas

---

Box 9.5 Situations where anticholinergic premedication may still be useful

As an antisialogogue
- During ketamine anaesthesia
- Awake fibreoptic intubation. Prevents dilution of local anaesthetic by saliva
- During surgery or instrumentation of the oral cavity, airway or oesophagus
- Planned inhalational induction of anaesthesia

For vagolytic effects on the heart
- During halothane anaesthesia, particularly induction in children
- Prior to suxamethonium, particularly in children
- Surgery in the territory of the trigeminal nerve

hyoscine has inhibitory (sedative and amnesic) effects. Both drugs have mild central antiemetic effects. Although disturbance of the CNS is not usually a problem at the doses used in anaesthetic premedication, some patients, particularly the elderly, may exhibit features of the central anticholinergic syndrome. These may include excitement, disorientation, hallucinations, ataxia, drowsiness, and even coma. Hyoscine has potent ocular effects and can cause prolonged blurred vision postoperatively. Glycopyrrolate (glycopyrronium bromide) is a quaternary amine and because of the resulting net positive charge, its hydrophilic molecule is unable to cross the blood–brain barrier. Glycopyrrolate therefore does not have any CNS side effects. It also causes less tachycardia and may therefore be preferable in patients with limited cardiovascular reserve.

The ratio of the relative potencies of atropine, hyoscine, and glycopyrrolate (as antisialogogues) is 1:2:3. The recommended doses for intramuscular premedication are 0.3–0.6 mg for atropine, 0.2–0.6 mg for hyoscine, and 0.2–0.4 mg for glycopyrrolate given 30–60 minutes preoperatively. However, atropine 2mg and hyoscine 1mg are also effective when given orally 90 minutes before surgery.[80] In the UK, hyoscine 0.3 mg is available without prescription for the treatment of motion sickness. Glycopyrrolate is poorly absorbed from the gastrointestinal tract because of its quaternary structure.

Antisympathomimetic effects
Sympathetic nervous activity is stimulated during laryngoscopy and tracheal intubation, surgery itself and emergence from anaesthesia. The resulting tachycardia and hypertension are undesirable in patients with ischaemic heart disease and poor left ventricular function. Untreated or uncontrolled hypertensive patients often exhibit extremes of both hypertension and hypotension during anaesthesia and surgery (rollercoastering or alpine anaesthesia).[81] Oral premedicant drugs can attenuate such responses, but it is preferable that surgery is postponed in patients with untreated or uncontrolled hypertension. Patients known to be hypertensive or with ischaemic heart disease should receive their usual medication up until surgery. The only exception to this is those patients taking angiotensin-converting enzyme (ACE) inhibitors for control of hypertension, which should be stopped the day before surgery. Continuation of ACE inhibitor therapy until the day of surgery is associated with an increased probability of hypotension at induction of anaesthesia.[82]

Oral β-blockers have been used effectively as premedicants.[83] They exert anxiolytic effects by antagonising circulating noradrenaline and adrenaline, thereby reducing the unwelcome physical symptoms and signs of anxiety such as tachycardia, palpitations, hypertension, and tremor. Similarly, they may be effective in attenuating the sympathetic responses to tracheal intubation and surgery, reducing the incidence of cardiac dysrhythmias and myocardial ischaemia[84-88]. Unlike the benzodiazepines, they are not sedative or amnesic and do not impair psychomotor performance.[89] However, β-blockers are not used routinely because, although they are effective in diminishing the above symptoms and signs of anxiety, they do not affect the psychological symptoms. Furthermore, their adverse side effects (bradycardia, atrioventricular conduction block, hypotension, bronchospasm, negative inotropy, and heart failure) may be potentiated by interactions with anaesthetic drugs.

Recently, premedication with selective α_2-adrenergic agonists has been shown to promote haemodynamic stability.[90-93] The most extensively studied drug is clonidine, which has been available for over 20 years to treat hypertension. Unlike the majority of hypotensive drugs, clonidine acts within both the central and peripheral nervous systems, causing presynaptic inhibition of noradrenaline release. The benefits of this dual action include anxiolysis, sedation, analgesia, a reduction in intraocular pressure and stabilisation of the cardiovascular system. Furthermore, there is a diminution in subsequent anaesthetic requirement, due to stimulation of central postsynaptic α_2-adrenoceptors. Clonidine is almost completely absorbed after oral administration and reaches peak plasma levels within 90 minutes. A dose of 200–300 μg is effective in producing satisfactory sedation and anxiolysis. Unfortunately, unwanted side effects, in particular dry mouth, oversedation and clinically relevant bradycardia and hypotension, have limited the adoption of clonidine as a routine premedicant. Dexmedetomidine, another α_2 agonist with greater selectivity and specificity, may prove to be more useful.

Premedication in special circumstances

Patients at risk of bacterial endocarditis

There are clear guidelines published in the *British National Formulary*[94] for the prevention of endocarditis in patients known to have a heart valve lesion (including mitral valve prolapse), prosthetic heart valve, septal defect or a patent ductus arteriosus. Patients with an undiagnosed heart murmur should be thoroughly questioned and examined to assess its importance and if necessary echocardiography should be performed. It is probably sensible to provide antibiotic prophylaxis for "innocent" murmurs in the absence of an echocardiographic diagnosis.

For most procedures it is recommended that antibiotics are given intravenously at induction of anaesthesia. However, amoxycillin 3 g may be given orally four hours before induction of anaesthesia for dental procedures to patients at risk, unless the patient has a prosthetic valve or a history of previous endocarditis.

Day surgery

Patients scheduled for day surgery may be particularly anxious as they have little time to acclimatise to the hospital environment although it has also been suggested that they are less anxious than other groups of patients.[95] Anxiolytic premedication is not routinely offered in the UK because of concerns over delayed recovery from anaesthesia and discharge from the day surgery unit. Oral temazepam and midazolam have the most appropriate profiles for day surgery premedication with both a rapid onset and short duration of action. Oral midazolam is not currently licensed in the UK.

Ischaemic heart disease

Patients with ischaemic heart disease should continue to receive their usual antianginal medication up to surgery. In addition, it is probably advisable to prescribe a topical glyceryl trinitrate (GTN) patch, applied the night before surgery, in patients who are still symptomatic and using sublingual GTN. If sedative premedication is prescribed, one should also consider giving the patient supplementary oxygen by face mask or nasal cannula.

Diabetes

Various strategies may be adopted depending on the usual method of control (diet, oral hypoglycaemics or insulin), the quality of control and the nature of the surgical procedure.[96] Patients whose diabetes is controlled by diet alone often do not require specific intervention, even for quite major surgery. Patients who take oral hypoglycaemic agents should have these discontinued at least the day before surgery and if necessary converted to intravenous insulin prior to surgery. All patients controlled with insulin, all poorly controlled diabetics and patients on oral hypoglycaemics having major surgery should be established on an intravenous insulin infusion at least the night before surgery. The Alberti regime in which 16 units of insulin are added to a 500 ml bag of 10% glucose containing 20 mmol of KCl running at 100 ml/h is a simple and effective means of achieving good control of peri-operative blood sugar.[97] However, this technique has now been largely superseded by the use of a variable-rate insulin infusion administered using an electronic syringe pump along with a separate glucose infusion. Frequent estimations of the blood glucose concentration determine the rate of insulin administration according to a predetermined scale.

Asthma

The patient's usual bronchodilator medication should be continued up to surgery. Some patients may benefit from nebulised salbutamol and/or

Atrovent given 1–2 hours before induction of anaesthesia. The use of preoperative corticosteroids should also be considered.

Paediatrics

There is no doubt that non-pharmacological approaches to anxiolysis are preferable when preparing children for anaesthesia and surgery. A sympathetic and friendly approach by ward staff, the anaesthetist, and surgeon is essential. The benefits of informal visits to the hospital ward and theatre complex before the day of surgery, so-called 'Saturday Clubs' and video presentations of what the child may typically expect have all been shown to be beneficial.[98] The importance of allowing parents to be present at induction of anaesthesia has similarly been proven effective in allaying anxiety of children,[83] although there are clearly situations when this approach may not be desirable.

However, some children will benefit from anxiolytic and sedative premedication. The most commonly prescribed drug for younger children in the UK is trimeprazine,[84] a sedating antihistamine with antiemetic properties. It is not particularly effective as an anxiolytic and if the sedative effect is not satisfactory, children may indeed exhibit agitation and distress. This has been more of a problem in recent years following the reduction in the recommended maximum dose (from 4 mg/kg to 1.5–2.0 mg/kg) due to several case reports involving postoperative cardiorespiratory collapse in children at the higher dose.[100] Oral midazolam syrup is widely used outside the UK and has been shown to be effective and well tolerated.[39,40] It is a better anxiolytic than trimeprazine and at a dose of 0.5 mg/kg tends to produce disinhibition and "drunkenness" rather than sedation. Although an unlicensed mode of administration, oral midazolam is in routine use in several hospitals in the UK. Older children above the age of about 10 years can be treated as young adults and given a benzodiazepine such as temazepam.

Topical EMLA cream and amethocaine gel are now used almost universally as premedicants in paediatric anaesthesia. They are both effective in reducing the pain of venous cannulation (and therefore also the fear of pain). EMLA must be applied at least one hour prior to anaesthesia whereas amethocaine gel is more rapidly absorbed into the dermis and is effective within 30 minutes. The introduction of topical anaesthesia has been one of the factors responsible for the transition from inhalational to intravenous induction of anaesthesia in children.

Pregnancy

During pregnancy, gastric acid secretion is increased. In late pregnancy, gastric emptying is also slowed, due to a number of factors including increased levels of progesterone and displacement of the pylorus by the enlarged uterus. During labour, pain, anxiety, and the administration of opioids further delay emptying. All of these factors prolong the time that solid food remains in the stomach after a meal. Furthermore, intragastric pressure is increased while at the same time, the lower oesophageal sphincter pressure is reduced, a situation exacerbated when opioids and anticholinergic drugs are administered. The net result of these changes is an increased risk of the patient regurgitating and aspirating during the induction of anaesthesia.

In order to reduce this risk, and that of pneumonitis should it occur, patients requiring operative delivery receive prophylactic treatment to reduce the volume and acidity of their gastric contents. Prior to elective caesarean section, patients are usually given two oral doses of ranitidine, 150 mg. The first dose is given the night before or eight hours prior to surgery and the second 1–2 hours before surgery. The second dose may be accompanied by metoclopramide. Finally, approximately 15 minutes before anaesthesia 0.3 M sodium citrate 30 ml is given orally. For emergency caesarean sections, there is not usually time for ranitidine to have a significant effect and therefore it is essential that a dose of sodium citrate is administered. However, a bolus of ranitidine 50 mg intravenously along with metoclopramide 10 mg are usually given for the beneficial effect they will have during recovery from anaesthesia when the risk of regurgitation is still high.

Atopy

The combination of preoperative H_1 and H_2 antagonists and corticosteroids may be useful in patients with a previous history of acute anaphylaxis, especially where the trigger has not been identified or cannot be avoided.

Patients taking oral corticosteroids

It has long been assumed that patients taking corticosteroids would have suffered supression of their hypothalamic-pituitary-adrenal (HPA) axis and be unable to respond to the stress of anaesthesia and surgery. This has generally resulted in the administration of prolonged or excessive supplementary doses of steroids in the perioperative period. This practice has continued despite awareness of the fact that excessive steroid administration is associated with a variety of adverse effects including delayed wound healing, immunosuppression, peptic ulceration, hyperglycaemia, electrolyte abnormalities, and psychological disturbances. Recently, a more rational approach to steroid therapy in the perioperative period has been suggested, based upon the normal response (Box 9.6).[101,102]

Acknowledgement

The authors would like to express their sincere thanks to Mrs Karen Gwinnutt for her expert help in preparing the manuscript for this chapter.

Box 9.6 Steroid therapy in the perioperative period[101,102]

- Patients taking less than 10 mg of prednisolone per day (or its equivalent) have a normal HPA axis and do not need any additional steroids.
- If it is more than three months since the patient last took steroids, then no steroids are required.
- If the patient is taking more than 10mg of prednisolone per day or has done so within the past three months, for all types of surgery the normal dose should be given preoperatively, then proceed as follows.
  - Minor surgery – if the above was omitted, give 25 mg hydrocortisone IV at induction and resume normal doses postoperatively.
  - Moderate surgery – 25 mg hydrocortisone IV at induction, followed by an IV infusion of 100 mg hydrocortisone over 24 hours. Normal doses can be resumed on the second day if there are no complications.
  - Major surgery – 25 mg hydrocortisone IV at induction, followed by an IV infusion of 100 mg hydrocortisone per 24 hours for 48–72 hours. Normal doses can be resumed when the gastrointestinal tract is functioning normally.
  - Patients taking immunosuppressant doses should be given their normal doses or the equivalent as hydrocortisone perioperatively. No additional doses are required.

---

1 Atkinson RS, Rushman GB, Lee JA. *A synopsis of anaesthesia*, 10th edn. Bristol:Wright, 1987.
2 Rushman GB, Davies NJH, Atkinson RS. *A short history of anaesthesia*. Oxford: Butterworth-Heinemann, 1996.
3 Mirakhur RK. Pre-anaesthetic medication: a survey of current usage. *J R Soc Med* 1991; 84: 481–3.
4 Alpert CC, Baker JD, Cooke JE. A rational approach to anaesthetic premedication. *Drugs* 1989; 37: 219–28.
5 Gwinnutt CL. *Clinical anaesthesia*. Oxford: Blackwell Science, 1996.
6 Madej TH, Paasuke RT. Anaesthetic premedication: aims, assessment and methods. *Can J Anaesth* 1987; 34: 259–73.
7 Guedel AE. *Inhalation anaesthesia*. New York: Macmillan, 1937.
8 Kanto J. Benzodiazepines as oral premedicants. *Br J Anaesth* 1981; 53: 1179–88.
9 Wallace LM. Psychological preparation as a method of reducing the stress of surgery. *J Human Stress* 1984; 10: 62–7.
10 Weiss OF, Sriwatanakul K, Weintraub M, Lasagna L. Reduction of anxiety and postoperative analgesic requirements by audiovisual instruction. *Lancet* 1983; 1: 43–4.
11 Johnston M. Anxiety in surgical patients. *Psychol Med* 1980; 10: 145–52.
12 Vogele C, Steptoe A. Physiological and subjective stress responses in surgical patients. *J Psychosom Res* 1986; 30: 205.
13 Egbert LD, Battit GE, Turndorf H, Beecher HK. The value of the preoperative visit by an anaesthetist. *JAMA* 1963; 185: 553–5.
14 Leigh JM, Walker J, Janaganathan P. Effect of preoperative anaesthetic visit on anxiety. *BMJ* 1977; ii: 987–9.
15 Lasagna L, von Felsinger JM, Beecher HK. Drug-induced mood changes in man. 1. Observations on healthy subjects, chronically ill patients and 'postaddicts'. *JAMA* 1955; 157: 1006–20.
16 Kanto J, Watanabe H, Namiki A. Pharmacological premedication for anaesthesia. *Acta Anaesthesiol Scand* 1996; 40: 982–90.
17 Wittenberg MI, Lark TL, Butler CL *et al.* Effects of oral diazepam on intravenous access in same day surgery patients. *J Clin Anesth* 1998; 10: 13–16.

18 Kontinen VK, Maunuksela EL, Sarvela J. Premedication with sublingual triazolam compared with oral diazepam. *Can J Anaesth* 1993; **40**: 829–34.
19 Pippingskold K, Lehtinen AM, Laatikainen T, Hanninen H, Korttila K. The effect of orally administered diazepam and midazolam on plasma beta-endorphin, ACTH and preoperative anxiety. *Acta Anaesthesiol Scand* 1991; **35**: 175–80.
20 Kirvela OA, Kanto JH. Clinical and metabolic responses to different types of premedication. *Anesth Analg* 1991; **73**: 49–53.
21 Ravnborg M, Hasselstrom L, Ostergard D. Premedication with oral and rectal diazepam. *Acta Anaesthesiol Scand* 1986; **30**: 132–8.
22 Pinnock CA, Fell D, Hunt PC, Miller R, Smith G. A comparison of triazolam and diazepam as premedication agents for minor gynaecological surgery. *Anaesthesia* 1985; **40**: 324–8.
23 Fry EN, Deshpande S. Oral premedication: diazepam, metoclopramide and a drink. *Anaesthesia* 1977; **32**: 370–2.
24 Fragen RJ, Caldwell N. Lorazepam premedication: lack of recall and relief of anxiety. *Anesth Analg* 1976; **55**: 792–6.
25 Thomas D, Tipping T, Halifax R, Blogg CE, Hollands MA. Triazolam premedication: a comparison with lorazepam and placebo in gynaecological patients. *Anaesthesia* 1986; **41**: 692–7.
26 van de Velde A, Camu F. Efficacy of lorazepam oral fast dissolving drug formulation (FDDF) in anesthesia premedication in adults: a double-blind placebo controlled comparison. *Acta Anaesthesiol Belg* 1988; **39**: 95–100.
27 Loach A, Fisher A. Lorazepam as a premedicant for day-case surgery: an assessment. *Anaesthesia* 1975; **30**: 545–9.
28 Aaltonen L, Kanto J, Salo M. Cerebrospinal fluid concentrations and serum protein binding of lorazepam and its conjugates. *Acta Pharmacol Toxicol* 1980; **46**: 156–8.
29 Turner GA, Paech M. A comparison of oral midazolam solution with temazepam as a day case premedicant. *Anaesth Intens Care* 1991; **19**: 365–8.
30 Ratcliff A, Indalo AA, Bradshaw EG, Rye RM. Premedication with temazepam in minor surgery. The relationship between plasma concentration and clinical effect after a dose of 40 mg. *Anaesthesia* 1989; **44**: 812–15.
31 Short TG, Galletly DC. Double-blind comparison of midazolam and temazepam as oral premedicants for outpatient anaesthesia. *Anaesth Intens Care* 1989; **17**: 151–6.
32 Hargreaves J. Benzodiazepine premedication in minor day-case surgery: comparison of oral midazolam and temazepam with placebo. *Br J Anaesth* 1988: **61**: 611–16.
33 Goroszeniuk T, Albin M, Jones RM, Mohamoud O. Pre-operative medication reviewed: oral temazepam compared with papaveretum and hyoscine. *Eur J Anaesthesiol* 1987; **4**: 261–7.
34 Kanto J. The use of oral benzodiazepines as premedications: the usefulness of temazepam. *Acta Psychiatr Scand* 1986; **332**(suppl): 159–66.
35 Lim TW, Thomas E, Choo SM. Premedication with midazolam is more effective by the sublingual than oral route. *Can J Anaesth* 1997; **44**: 723–6.
36 McCluskey A, Meakin G. Oral administration of midazolam as a premedicant for paediatric day-case anaesthesia. *Anaesthesia* 1994; **49**: 782–5.
37 Patel D, Meakin G. Oral midazolam compared with diazepam-droperidol and trimeprazine as premedicants in children. *Paed Anaesth* 1997; **7**: 287–93.
38 Kortilla K, Aromaa U, Tammisto T. Patient's expectations and acceptance of the effects of the drugs given before anaesthesia: comparison of light and amnesic premedication. *Acta Anaesthesiol Scand* 1981; **25**: 381–6.
39 Payne KA, Coetzee AR, Mattheyse FJ, Heydenrych JJ. Behavioural changes in children following minor surgery – is premedication beneficial? *Acta Anaesthesiol Belg* 1992; **43**: 173–9.
40 McQuay HJ. Pre-emptive analgesia: a systematic review of clinical studies. *Ann Med* 1995; **27**: 249–56.
41 Kortilla K. The study of postoperative nausea and vomiting. *Br J Anaesth* 1992; **69** (suppl 1): 20S–23S.
42 Albibi R, McCallum RW. Metoclopramide: pharmacology and clinical application. *Ann Intern Med* 1983; **98**: 86–95.

181

43 Proctor JD, Chremos AN, Evans EF, Wasserman AJ. An apomorphine-induced vomiting model for antiemetic studies in man. *J Clin Pharmacol* 1978; **18**: 95–9.

44 Elliott RH, Graham SG, Curran JP. Sustained release metoclopramide for prophylaxis of postoperative nausea and vomiting. *Eur J Anaesthesiol* 1994; **11**: 465–7.

45 Malins AF, Field JM, Nesling PM, Cooper GM. Nausea and vomiting after gynaecological laparoscopy: comparison of premedication with oral ondansetron, metoclopramide and placebo. *Br J Anaesth* 1994; **72**: 231–3.

46 Kymer PJ, Brown RE, Lawhorn CD, Jones E, Pearce L. The effects of oral droperidol versus oral metoclopramide versus both oral droperidol and metoclopramide on postoperative vomiting when used as a premedicant for strabismus surgery. *J Clin Anesth* 1995; **7**: 35–9.

47 Nicolson SC, Kaya KM, Betts EK. The effect of preoperative oral droperidol on the incidence of postoperative emesis after paediatric strabismus surgery. *Can J Anaesth* 1988; **35**: 364–7.

48 Madej TH, Simpson KH. Comparison of the use of domperidone, droperidol and metoclopramide in the prevention of nausea and vomiting following major gynaecological surgery. *Br J Anaesth* 1986; **58**: 884–7.

49 Jellish WS, Leonetti JP, Fluder E, Thalji Z. Ondansetron versus droperidol or placebo to prevent nausea and vomiting after otologic surgery. *Otolaryngol Head Neck Surg* 1998; **118**: 785–9.

50 Sniadach MS, Alberts MS. A comparison of the prophylactic antiemetic effect of ondansetron and droperidol on patients undergoing gynecologic laparoscopy. *Anesth Analg* 1997; **85**: 797–800.

51 Stienstra R, Samhan YM, el-Mofty M, de Bont LE, Bovill JG. Double-blind comparison of alizapride, droperidol and ondansetron in the treatment of postoperative nausea. *Eur J Anaesthesiol* 1997; **14**: 290–4.

52 Fujii Y, Tanaka H, Toyooka H. Preoperative oral granisetron prevents postoperative nausea and vomiting. *Acta Anaesthesiol Scand* 1998; **42**: 653–7.

53 Fujii Y, Saitoh Y, Tanaka H, Toyooka H. Prevention of PONV with granisetron, droperidol or metoclopramide in patients with postoperative emesis. *Can J Anaesth* 1998; **45**: 153–6.

54 Fujii Y, Tanaka H, Toyooka H. Prevention of nausea and vomiting in female patients undergoing breast surgery: a comparison with granisetron, droperidol, metoclopramide and placebo. *Acta Anaesthesiol Scand* 1998; **42**: 220–4.

55 Fujii Y, Tanaka H, Toyooka H. Prevention of postoperative nausea and vomiting with a combination of granisetron and droperidol. *Anesth Analg* 1998; **86**: 613–16.

56 Alexander R, Fennelly M. Comparison of ondansetron, metoclopramide and placebo as premedicants to reduce nausea and vomiting after major surgery. *Anaesthesia* 1997; **52**: 695–8.

57 Rust M, Cohen LA. Single oral dose ondansetron in the prevention of postoperative nausea and emesis. *Anaesthesia* 1994; **49**(suppl): 16–23.

58 Leeser J, Lip H. Prevention of postoperative nausea and vomiting using ondansetron, a new, selective 5-HT3 receptor antagonist. *Anesth Analg* 1991; **72**: 751–5.

59 Figuerado ED, Canosa LG. Ondansetron in the prophylaxis of postoperative vomiting: a meta-analysis. *J Clin Anesth* 1998; **10**: 211–21.

60 Tarkkila P, Torn K, Tuominen M, Lindgren L. Premedication with promethazine and transdermal scopolamine reduces the incidence of nausea and vomiting after intrathecal morphine. *Acta Anaesthesiol Scand* 1995; **39**: 983–6.

61 Thune A, Appelgren L, Haglind E. Prevention of postoperative nausea and vomiting after laparoscopic cholecystectomy. A prospective randomized study of metoclopramide and transdermal hyoscine. *Eur J Surg* 1995; **161**: 265–8.

62 Koski EM, Mattila MA, Knapik D *et al.* Double blind comparison of transdermal hyoscine and placebo for the prevention of postoperative nausea. *Br J Anaesth* 1990; **64**: 16–20.

63 Wilkinson AR, Frampton CM, Glover PW, Davis FM. Preoperative transdermal hyoscine for the prevention of postoperative nausea and vomiting. *Anaesth Intens Care* 1989; **17**: 285–9.

64 Uppington J, Dunnet J, Blogg CE. Transdermal hyoscine and postoperative nausea and vomiting. *Anaesthesia* 1986; **41**: 16–20.

65 Pandit SK, Kothary SP, Pandit UA, Mirakhur RK. Premedication with cimetidine and metoclopramide. Effect on the risk factors of acid aspiration. *Anaesthesia* 1986; **41**: 486–92.

66 Sutherland AD, Maltby JR, Sale JP, Reid CR. The effect of preoperative oral fluid and ranitidine on gastric fluid volume and pH. *Can J Anaesth* 1987; **34**: 117–21.

67 Aromaa U, Kalima TV. Ranitidine and prevention of pulmonary aspiration syndrome. *Acta Anaesthesiol Scand* 1986; **30**: 10–12.

68 Jacobs BR, Swift CA, Dubow HD *et al.* Time required for oral ranitidine to decrease gastric fluid acidity. *Anesth Analg* 1991; **73**: 787–9.

69 Vila P, Espachs P, Echevarria V, Garcia M, Rincon R, Vidal F. Acid aspiration prophylaxis in elective biliary surgery. A comparison of omeprazole and famotidine using manually aided gastric aspiration. *Anaesthesia* 1994; **49**: 909–11.

70 Escolano F, Castano J, Pares N, Bisbe E, Monterde J. Comparison of the effects of famotidine and ranitidine on gastric secretion in patients undergoing elective surgery. *Anaesthesia* 1989; **44**: 212–15.

71 Gallagher EG, White M, Ward S, Contrell J, Mann SG. Prophylaxis against acid aspiration syndrome. Single oral dose of H_2-antagonist on the evening before elective surgery. *Anaesthesia* 1988; **43**: 1011–14.

72 Ewart MC, Yau G, Gin T, Kotur CF, Oh TE. A comparison of the effects of omeprazole and ranitidine on gastric secretion in women undergoing elective caesarean section. *Anaesthesia* 1990; **45**: 527–30.

73 Escolano F, Castano J, Lopez R, Bisbe E, Alcon A. Effects of omeprazole, ranitidine, famotidine and placebo on gastric secretion in patients undergoing elective surgery. *Br J Anaesth* 1992; **69**: 404–6.

74 Nishina K, Mikawa K, Maekawa N, Takao Y, Shiga M, Obara H. A comparison of lansoprazole, omeprazole and ranitidine for reducing preoperative gastric secretion in adult patients undergoing elective surgery. *Anesth Analg* 1996; **82**: 832–6.

75 Yau G, Kan AF, Gin T, Oh TE. A comparison of omeprazole and ranitidine for prophylaxis against aspiration pneumonitis in emergency caesarian section. *Anaesthesia* 1992; **47**: 101–4.

76 Kluger MT, Owen H, Plummer JL, McLean C. The effect of oral cisapride premedication on fasting gastric volumes. *Anaesth Intens Care* 1995; **23**: 687–90.

77 Rowbotham DJ, Bamber PA, Nimmo WS. Comparison of the effect of cisapride and metoclopramide on morphine-induced delay in gastric emptying. *Br J Clin Pharmacol* 1988; **26**: 741–6.

78 Lim SK, Elegbe EO. Ranitidine and sodium citrate as prophylaxis against acid aspiration syndrome in obstetric patients undergoing caesarian section. *Singapore Med J* 1992; **33**: 608–10.

79 Mirakhur RK, Clarke RSJ, Dundee JW, McDonald JR. Anticholinergic drugs in anaesthesia: a survey of their present position. *Anaesthesia* 1978; **33**: 133–8.

80 Mirakhur RK. Comparative study of the effects of oral and i.m. atropine and hyoscine in volunteers. *Br J Anaesth* 1978; **50**: 591–8.

81 Prys-Roberts C, Meloche R, Foëx P. Studies of anaesthesia in relation to hypertension. 1: Cardiovascular responses of treated and untreated patients. *Br J Anaesth* 1971; **43**: 122–37.

82 Smith MS, Muir H, Hall R. Perioperative management of drug therapy. Clinical considerations. *Drugs* 1996; **51**: 238–59.

83 Jakobsen CJ, Blom L. Preoperative assessment of anxiety and measurement of arterial plasma catecholamine concentrations. The effect of oral beta-adrenergic blockade with metoprolol. *Anaesthesia* 1989; **44**: 249–52.

84 Davies MJ, Dysart RH, Silbert BS, Scott DA, Cook RJ. Prevention of tachycardia with atenolol pretreatment for carotid endarterectomy under cervical plexus blockade. *Anaesth Intens Care* 1992; **20**: 161–4.

85 Whitehead MH, Whitmarsh VB, Horton JN. Metoprolol in anaesthesia for oral surgery. The effect of pretreatment on the incidence of cardiac dysrhythmias. *Anaesthesia* 1980; **35**: 779–82.

86 Jakobsen CJ, Blom L, Brondbjerg M, Lenler-Petersen P. Effect of metoprolol and diazepam on preoperative anxiety. *Anaesthesia* 1990; **45**: 40–3.

87 Hanna MH, Heap DG, Kimberley AP. Cardiac dysrhythmia associated with general anaesthesia for oral surgery. Its prevention by the prophylactic use of an oral beta-adrenergic blocker. *Anaesthesia* 1983; **38**: 1192–4.

88 Stone JG, Foëx P, Sear JW, Johnson LL, Khambatta HJ, Triner L. Myocardial ischaemia in untreated hypertensive patients: effect of a single small oral dose of a beta-adrenergic blocking agent. *Anesthesiology* 1988; **68**: 495–500.

89 Betts TA, Knight R, Crowe A, Blake A, Harvey P, Mortiboy D. Effect of beta-blockers on psychomotor performance in normal volunteers. *Eur J Clin Pharmacol* 1985; **28**(suppl): 39–49.

90 Sanderson PM, Eltringham R. The role of clonidine in anaesthesia. *Hosp Med* 1998; **59**: 221–3.

91 Laurito CE, Baughman VL, Becker GL, Desilva TW, Carranza CJ. The effectiveness of oral clonidine as a sedative/anxiolytic and as a drug to blunt the hemodynamic responses to laryngoscopy. *J Clin Anesth* 1991; **3**: 186–93.

92 Wright PM, Carabine UA, McClune S, Orr DA, Moore J. Preanaesthetic medication with clonidine. *Br J Anaesth* 1990; **65**: 628–32.

93 Pouttu J, Scheinin B, Rosenberg PH, Viinamaki O, Scheinin M. Oral premedication with clonidine: effects on stress responses during general anaesthesia. *Acta Anaesthesiol Scand* 1987; **31**: 730–4.

94 British Medical Association and the Royal Pharmaceutical Society of Great Britain. *British National Formulary no 35*. London: British Medical Association and the Royal Pharmaceutical Society of Great Britain, 1998.

95 Male CG. Anxiety in day surgery patients. *Br J Anaesth* 1981; **53**: 663P.

96 Peters A, Kerner W. Perioperative management of the diabetic patient. *Exp Clin Endocrinol Diabetes* 1995; **103**: 213–18.

97 Thomas DJ, Platt HS, Alberti KG. Insulin-dependent diabetes during the perioperative period. An assessment of continuous glucose-insulin-potassium infusion and traditional treatment. *Anaesthesia* 1984; **39**: 629–37.

98 Vernon DT, Bailey WC. Use of motion pictures in psychologically preparing children for induction of anesthesia. *Anesthesiology* 1974; **40**: 68–72.

99 Schulman JL, Foley JM, Vernon DTA, Allan D. A study of the effect of the mother's presence during anaesthesia induction. *Paediatrics* 1967; **39**: 111–14.

100 Loan WB, Cuthbert D. Adverse cardiovascular response to oral trimeprazine in children. *BMJ* 1985; **290**: 1548–9.

101 Nicholson G, Burrin JM, Hall GM. Peri-operative steroid supplementation. *Anaesthesia* 1998; **53**: 1091–104.

102 Anon. Drugs in the perioperative period 2 – Corticosteroids and therapy for diabetes mellitus. *Drug Ther Bull* 1999; **37**: 68–70.

Epilogue

Now this is not the end.
It is not even the beginning of the end.
But it is, perhaps, the end of the beginning.

Winston Churchill

Any book devoted to assessment and preparation of the patient for anaesthesia and surgery must acknowledge what follows in the operating theatre. Safe anaesthesia is the result of prior planning, preparation and choice of appropriate anaesthetic technique together with a thorough understanding of the proposed surgical procedure. What the authors of the preceding chapters have tried to emphasise is that careful preparation of the patient for anaesthesia and surgery will reduce the likelihood of the patient coming to harm. Inevitably the anaesthetic itself may have an influence on outcome. However, the choice of appropriate anaesthetic technique is beyond the scope of the present book and is the subject of numerous other reputable anaesthetic texts. Nevertheless, if this book has made the reader more aware of the crucial importance of preoperative patient evaluation then both the editor and the authors will have achieved their aim.

Index

α_2 adrenergic agonists 176
α_2-adrenoceptor antagonists 12
α-adrenergic receptor blockade 112
abdominal system 29–30
ACE inhibitors 12–13, 98, 102, 175
acetylcholine receptors 128
acid aspiration 172
acidosis 21
activated partial thromboplastin time
    (aPTT) 51, 122
acute asthma 63
acute hepatitis 119
acute renal failure (ARF) 31
acute tubular necrosis (ATN) 119
Addison's disease 32, 111
adrenal disease 52, 111–13
adrenaline 98
adrenocortical dysfunction 32, 111–12
adrenocorticotrophic hormone
    (ACTH) 111, 112
adverse events, perioperative period
    80
age, and anxiety 10
airway assessment 28
Alberti regime 177
albumin 114, 120
alcohol abuse 66
alimentary tract 65–6
American College of Cardiology 47,
    94
American College of Physicians 85
American Heart Association 47
American Society of Anesthesiologists
    (ASA) 8, 58, 59, 83, 159–60
amethocaine 178
aminoglycosides 73
amiodarone 99, 100
amnesia 169
amoxycillin 176
anaemia 50, 67, 118, 120–1, 125
anaesthetists

assessment by 8–9
    preoperative visits 4
analgesia 33, 166, 170
analgesics 73
angina 59, 97
angiotensin-converting enzyme *see* ACE
    inhibitors
ankylosing spondylitis 68
antacids 13, 117, 125, 159, 172–4
antiarrhythmics 13
antiautonomic effects 174–6
antibiotics 73, 111
anticholinergics 104, 106, 128, 159,
    174–5
anticholinesterases 128
anticoagulants 13, 123–4
antidiabetic therapy 13
antidiuretic hormone (ADH) 113, 114
antiemesis 22, 170–2
antihistamine 178
antiinflammatory agents 33, 103
antiplatelet drugs 13
antisympathomimetic effects 175–6
antithyroids 110
anxiety 10–12
anxiolysis 12, 166–9
anxiolytics 165
aortic regurgitation 101
aortic stenosis 101
aortocaval compression 69
apnoea 64
apomorphine 156
arachidonic acid 103
arrhythmias 73, 98–101, 113, 114, 115,
    173
arteriosclerosis 118
arthritis 33, 67–8, 69
arthrodesis 68
ascites 31, 119–20
aspiration 29–30, 61, 149, 150, 151,
    152, 154–8, 172, 173

aspirin 97, 119, 124
assessments *see* preoperative
    assessments; risk assessment
asthma
    implications 62–3, 69
    premedication 177–8
    preoperative optimisation 102–5
atelectasis 61, 150
atenolol 96
atlantoaxial instability 68
atopy 179
atrial fibrillation 24, 100
atrioventricular (AV) conduction
    defects 99
atropine 98, 108, 128, 159, 164, 174–5
Atrovent 178
Audit Commision 4–5
autoimmune disease 69
automation, preoperative screening 7
autonomic neuropathy 32, 107–8,
    155–6
azathioprine 128

β_2-adrenoceptor antagonists 12
β_2-agonists 103, 104, 106
β-blockade 65
β-blockers 96, 97, 98, 100, 101, 110,
    112, 167, 175–6
bacterial endocarditis 118, 176
barbiturates 166
Bayes' theorem 82
Bayesian model 82
benzodiazepines 73, 165, 166, 167, 170
biguanides 32, 108
bleeding disorders 22, 30, 123
blood pressure 26, 101
blood sugar 32, 52, 64, 108, 109, 153
blood urea nitrogen 52
blood volume abnormalities 126
body mass index 30
Bolam case 136
bowel obstruction 66
bradyarrhythmias 98
bradycardia 98, 107
brain abscesses 71
breast milk 157–8
breathlessness 23
broad-complex tachycardias 99

bronchodilators 13, 50, 103, 104, 177
bronchospasm 50, 61, 63, 105
bruising 51
bullous disease 64
bupivacaine 173
burns 34
butyrophenone 171

C-reactive protein 45
calcitonin 114, 115
calcium channel blockers 13, 72, 101
calcium gluconate 115
calcium salts 73
carbamazepine 173
carbidopa 127
carbimazole 110
carboxyhaemoglobin 106
carcinoid syndrome 66
cardiac disease 15, 69
cardiac murmurs 25, 46
cardiac performance 45–6
cardiac rhythm 45
cardiac risk indices 84–6
cardiac tamponade 68
cardiomegaly 46, 111
cardiomyopathies 29, 66, 67, 69, 97
Cardiopulmonary Risk Index (CPRI)
    87
cardiovascular disease
    implications 59–60
    preoperative optimisation 94–102
cardiovascular disturbances
    dialysis patients 126
    liver disease 118
cardiovascular system
    assessment 44–9
    examination 24–6
    history 22–4
cardioversion 100
catecholamines 112, 113, 166
central nervous system (CNS) 29, 70–1
cerebral arterial disease 71
cerebral oedema 113, 114
cerebrovascular disease 71
Chatterton v Gerson 135
chest pain 23
chest radiographs (CXR) 50
Child-Pugh classification 117, *118*

children
parental consent 142–3
premedication 178
preoperative assessments 15
respiratory tract infection 63–4
risk of aspiration 157–8
chlordiazepoxide 167
chloroform 164
chlorpropamide 108
chronic anaemia 67
chronic hepatitis 66
chronic obstructive pulmonary disease
(COPD) 61, 105
chronic renal failure (CRF) 31, 127
cimetidine 173
cirrhosis 31, 118, 119, 120
cisapride 159, 173
claudication 24
clinics, preanaesthetic 6–7
clonidine 176
coagulation
assessments 50–1
dialysis patients 125
disorders 122–5
coagulopathies 22, 30–1, 117–18,
122–3
coma 113
compliance, consent by 136
conduction disturbances 98, 99
Confidential Enquiry into Perioperative
Deaths (CEPOD) 58
congenital coagulation disorders 124–5
congestive heart failure (CHF) 45–6,
97–8, 100, 110, 118
Conn's syndrome 112
consent 133–47
decision plan 145–7
evidence of 135–6
informed 42–3, 136–8
mental incapacity 139–41
premedication 142–3
sectionalised 138–9
surgery 143–4
withholding 135
consent forms 135–6
consultants, working with 48–9
convulsions 113, 114, 115
coping behaviour 12

coronary artery bypass graft (CABG)
96–7
coronary artery disease (CAD) 94–7,
100, 107
coronary artery stenting 85
Coronary Artery Surgery Study
(CASS) 86
coronary vasospasm 106
corticosteroids 70, 103, 104, 106, 128,
178, 179
cortisol 111
coughs 27
creatinine 31, 52, 119, 127
cricoid pressure 30
Crohn's disease 12
cryoprecipitate 123, 124, 125
Cushing's syndrome 32, 111, 112
cyanosis 28, 150
cytochrome P-450 173

dalteparin 24
dantrolene 22
day surgery 16, 29, 177
deaths
anaesthetic 79, 149
perioperative 58
decision plans, consent 145–7
defensive testing 42
dehydration 152
dementia 29
depression 71
desmethyldiazepam 168
desmopressin 114, 124, 125
dexmedetomidine 176
deyhydration 122
diabetes insipidus 114
diabetes mellitus 69, 97
implications 64–5
premedication 177
preoperative assessment 31–2, 44
preoperative optimisation 107–9
diagnostic sticks 64
dialysis patients 125–6
diamorphine 98
Diazemuls 168
diazepam 167–8, 173
diclofenac 31
digoxin 13, 100

diltiazem 100
disseminated intravascular coagulation
    (DIC) 123
diuresis 115, 119
diuretics 33, 52, 73, 98, 102, 114, 115,
    127
dobutamine 98
doctors, preoperative assessments 7–8
doctrine of informed consent 137
dopamine 71, 127
dopexamine 98
Dormicum 169
Down's syndrome 68
droperidol 167, 171
drug history 22
drug therapy 93
drugs, perioperative period 12–13
dysarthria 29
dysphagia 29
dysphoria 167
dyspnoea 27, 28, 50, 150
dysrhythmias 69, 166
dystrophies 29, 70

echocardiography (ECHO) 46
education 14
Eisenmenger's syndrome 69
elderly patients 5, 29, 33
elective surgery 14–16
electroconvulsive treatment (ECT) 71
electrolyte disturbances
    dialysis patients 126
    preoperative assessment 52–3
    preoperative optimisation 113–15,
        120
electrolyte losses 116–17
emergency patients, aspiration 156–7
emergency surgery 16–17, 60
EMLA cream 178
encephalitis 71
encephalopathy 120
endocarditis 118, 176
endocrine disease
    implications 64–5
    preoperative assessment 52–3
    preoperative optimisation 107–15
endocrine system 31–2
ephedrine 98, 108

epilepsy 29, 70
epinephrine 98, 108
erythropoietin 125
esmolol 110
ether 164
ethics, of investigations 42–4
evaluation, of risks 81
exophthalmos 32

factor VIII 123, 124
family history 21–2
Family Law Reform Act 143
famotidine 173
fasting see preoperative fasting
fears 10–12
ferrous sulphate 120
fibrin 122
fibrinogen 122, 123
flecainide 100
fluid losses 116
fluids 161
flumazenil 167
forced expiratory volume (FEV) 61,
    102
forced vital capacity (FVC) 61, 102
Fragmin 24
frusemide 115, 119, 120, 127
functional impairment, assessment 93

gastric emptying 65, 150, 158–9
gastric PH, promoting 159
gastric physiology, pharmocology
    158–9
gastrin 151, 155
gastro-oesophageal disease 156
gastro-oesophageal reflux 150, 155,
    156, 157
gastrointestinal disease
    implications 65–6
    preoperative optimisation 115–17
gastrokinetic agents 13, 173
General Medical Council 133
Glasgow Coma Scale 29, 30
glibenclamide 32, 108
gliclazide 32
glottic oedema 155
glucocorticoids 103, 111, 112, 115
glucometers 64

glucose 32, 52, 108, 109, 114, 153
glyceryl trinitrate 98, 177
glycopyrrolate 159, 175
Goldman Cardiac Risk Index 83, 84, 85, 87
gravid uterus 154–5
Guillain-Barré syndrome 70

H₂ receptor antagonists 117
haematocrit 50–1, 121, 125
haematological disease, preoperative optimisation 120–5
haematology, assessments 50–1
haemodialysis 119
haemoglobin 50–1, 120
haemoglobinopathies 121–2
haemophilia A 122, 124
haemorrhagic cerebrovascular disease 71
haemostatic abnormalities 122–5
headaches 112
Health and Safety Executive 79–80
HealthQuiz 7, 41
heart block 24
heart failure 23, 25, 36, 59, 65, 111
heartburn 29, 65
HELLP syndrome 69
heparin 122, 123
hepatic cirrhosis 31
hepatic function 52
hepatic system 30–1
hepatitis 31, 66, 119, 126
hepatoma 119
hepatorenal syndrome 66, 119
hiatus hernia 29, 117
His-Purkinje fibres 68
histamine 63
histamine H₂ blockers 30
histamine receptor antagonists 125, 159, 173
hormone therapy 13
Hospital Anxiety and Depression (HAD) Scale 11
House of Lords 137
human immuno-deficiency virus (HIV) 43–4
humidification 106
hydration 115

hydrocortisone 111, 112
5-hydroxytryptamine 66
hyoscine 159, 164–5, 172, 174, 175
hyperaldosteronism 112
hypercalcaemia 114–15
hypercarbia 21, 103, 111
hypercholesterolaemia 44, 45
hypercoagulability 97
hyperglycaemia 64, 113
hyperkalaemia 73, 112, 114, 126, 129
hypernatraemia 114
hyperosmolality 122
hyperprexia 21–2
hypertension 32, 97, 107, 112, 166
implications 59–60, 64, 69
preoperative assessment 15, 25–6
preoperative optimisation 101–2
hyperthermia 129
hyperthyroidism 110
hypertonic hyponatraemia 113
hypertonicity 70
hypnotics 73
hypocalcaemia 115
hypoglycaemia 31, 64, 108, 109, 152, 153
hypokalaemia 33, 53, 99, 100, 114, 115, 120
hypomagnesaemia 115
hyponatraemia 112, 113, 120
hypoparathyroidism 32, 115
hypophosphataemia 115
hypotension 95, 102, 107, 111
hypothyroidism 32, 110–11
hypotonic hyponatraemia 113
hypoventilation 61
hypovolaemia 26, 112, 118, 122, 126
hypovolaemic hyponatraemia 113
hypoxaemia 31, 61, 105
hypoxia 63, 100, 103, 105, 111, 119, 121

immunosuppression 33, 128
incompetent adults, consent 140–1
indomethacin 119
infections
CNS 71
dialysis patients 126
respiratory tract 63–4, 105

informatics 41
information, excessive 11–12
informed consent 42–3, 136–8
inodilators 98
insulin 32, 73, 108, 109, 114, 177
intercurrent disease 58–73
interventricular conduction defects 99
intestinal obstruction 115–17
intubation 28, 61
invasive assessment 48
invasive monitoring 96
irritability 152, 153
ischaemic heart disease 32, 46–8, 64,
    97, 113, 118, 177
isoprenaline 24, 98
isoproterenol 98
isotonic hyponatraemia 113
isovolaemic hyponatraemia 113

jaundice 66, 119
Jehovah's Witnesses 15–16
juvenile chronic arthritis 33
juvenile rheumatoid arthritis 68

K⁺ ion concentration 70
kayexalate enemas 114
ketoacidosis 32, 109, 126

l-thyroxine 111
lactic acidosis 108
lactulose 120
laryngeal stridor 115
laryngoscopy 65
laryngospasm 61, 151
    12-lead electrocardiogram (ECG)
    45, 47
leukotriene antagonists 103
levodopa 127
lignocaine 99, 101
    5-lipoxygenase 103
lithium 73
liver 52
liver disease
  implications 66
  preoperative optimisation 117–20
lorazepam 168
lung disease 64, 86

magnesium 73, 109, 115, 126
magnesium trisilicate 159
malaise 152, 153
Mallampati's technique 28
mannitol 127
masive transfusion 122–3
mathematical modelling 81–2
Maxolon 168
medical conditions 5
Mendelson's syndrome 172
meningitis 71
Mental Health Act 140
mental incapacity, consent 139–41
metabolic abnormalities 52–3
metabolic control 108–9
metformin 32, 108
metoclopramide 156, 168, 171, 173
metodopramide 158–9
microthrombi 97
midazolam 169, 173, 177, 178
migraine 70
mineralcorticoids 111
mithramycin 115
mitral stenosis 101
Mobitz second-degree block 99
montelukast 104
morbidity
  aspiration 152
  CHF 45
  diabetics 64
  preoperative conditions 36
  respiratory disease 87
morphine 31, 164, 170, 173
mortality
  diabetics 64
  emergency surgery 60
  encephalopathy 120
  heart failure 36
  hypertension 60
  out of hours operating 81
motor neurone disease 29
Multiple Affect Adjective Checklist
    (MAACL) 11
multiple extrasystoles 24
multiple logistic regression 82
multiple regression 82
multiple sclerosis 29, 71, 129
multivariate analysis 82

muscle relaxants 29, 73, 165
muscle wasting 29
muscular dystrophy 70
musculoskeletal system 33
myasthenia gravis 29, 70, 128
myeloma 113
myocardial infarction 59, 60, 85, 96–7
myocardium 95, 97, 110
myopathies 29
myotonia 70
myxoedema coma 111

narrow-complex tachycardias 99–100
nasogastric tubes 116, 156
nausea, postoperative 22
NCEPOD report 4, 81
needle phobia 72
needlestick injury 31
neomycin 120
neostigmine 128
nephropathy 32, 107
nephrotoxic drugs 31
nerve degeneration 70
neuroleptics 167
neurological diseases 29, 69
    implications 70–1
    preoperative optimisation 127–9
neuromuscular diseases 29
neuropathies 32, 65, 70, 107–8, 155–6
New York Heart Association 23
nicotine 106
nifedipine 72, 101
nil-by-mouth 152
nitrogylcerine 96
nitrous oxide 165
non-insulin dependent diabetes
    mellitus (NDDM) 31–2, 108
non-invasive stress tests 48
non-steroidal antiinflammatory drugs
    (NSAIDs) 123–4
normothermia 111
normovolaemic anaemia 50
nurses, preoperative assessments 7
nutrition
    liver disease 120
    peripheral neuropathies 70
    preoperative assessments 12

obesity 12, 155–6
occipital cervical fusion 68
occlusive cerebrovascular disease 71
occupational disorders 21
oesophageal varices 118
oestrogen 125
oliguria 26, 69
omeprazole 159, 173
Omnopon 165
ondansetron 171
operations, NCEPOD classification 17
opiates 65
opioids 165, 167, 170
orthopnoea 50
osmolality 113
osteoporosis 33
our of hours operating 81
oxygen 96, 97, 98, 118, 165

pacemakers 24, 99
paediatrics see children
palpitations 24
panels, of tests 51
paracentesis 119
parental consent 142–3
Parkinson's disease 70, 71, 127
Parsonnet Risk Index 83
partial thromboplastin time (PTT) 42,
    51, 122
pathophysiology 150–1
patients
    anxiety and fears 10–12
    consent see consent
    on dialysis 125–6
    preoperative assessments 35–8
peak expiratory flow rate (PEFR) 102
Pearce v United Bristol Healthcare
    NHST [1999] PIQR53 138
penicillamine 33
pepsin 151
percutaneous transluminal angioplasty
    85
pericardial effusions 111
perioperative optimisation 93–129
peripheral nervous system 70
peripheral oedema 46, 69
phaeochromocytoma 52, 112–13
pharmocological considerations 72–3

pharmocology, gastric physiology 158–9
phenotypes 22
phenoxybenzamine 112, 113
phenytoin 173
phosphate 115
physical status 37, 58, 59, 83–4
physical therapies 93
physiology 150–1
physiotherapy 106, 119
plasma 118
plasma ammonia 120
plasma cholinesterase (Pche) deficiency
    22
plasmapheresis 128
plasminogen activator 124, 125
platelets 51
pleural effusions 111, 119
pneumonia 61, 105, 173
pneumonitis 151, 152, 179
pneumothorax 107
polycythaemia 50
polyuria 112
postoperative nausea and vomiting
    (PONV) 170
postpartum haemorrhage 69
potassium 22, 29, 53, 73, 99, 109, 113,
    114, 120
potassium iodide 110
prazosin 112
predictive models 82
predictive respiratory complication
    quotient (PRQ) 87
prednisolone 111
preeclampsia 69
pregnancy
    implications 68–9
    premedication 178–9
    risk of aspiration 154–5
    testing for 43
premature ventricular contractions
    (PVCs) 100
premedication 164–80
    aims of 165–76
    consent 142–3
    gastric contents 152
    special circumstances 176–9
preoperative assessments
    cardiovascular system 44–9

coagulation 50–1
conducting 7–9
haematology 50–1
history and examination 21–34
methods of 6–7
patients 35–8
pulmonary system 50
serum biochemistry 51–3
preoperative fasting
    guidelines 159–61
    history 149–50
    normal population 151–4
    physiology and pathophysiology
        150–1
    promoting gastric emptying 158–9
    promoting gastric pH 159
    risk of aspiration 154–8
preoperative testing
    developing a rationale 38–9
    ethics of investigations 42–4
    evaluating test performance 39–41
    follies 42
    informatics 41
    optimisation of 53–5
    routine 36
preoperative tests, under-ordering of 53
preoperative visits
    current practice 3–5
    screening versus assessment 5–7
prior predictive value 40–1
probability inference 82
procainamide 100
prokinetics 117, 156, 158–9
propranolol 110, 112, 113, 173
propylthiouracil 110
prostaglandins 119
prothrombin time (PT) 42, 51, 118,
    122
proton pump inhibitors 117, 159, 173
psychiatric disease, implications 71–2
psychological considerations 71–2
psychological preparation 9–12
pulmonary disturbances, liver disease
    119
pulmonary function tests (PFTs) 50
pulmonary oedema 67
pulmonary risk indices 86–8
pulmonary system, assessments 50

pulmonary *x* rays 50
pyrexia 63
pyridostigmine 128

Q waves 47
questionnaires 6, *10*
Quetelet's index 30

radial arteries 26
rales 46
ranitidine 30, 159, 173, 174, 179
reactive airway disease 102
records, risk assessments 81
red blood cell transfusion 121
referrals 7
reflux 150, 155, 156, 157
regurgitation 65, 101, 149, 150, 152, 156
renal disease
  implications 66–7
  preoperative optimisation 125–7
renal disturbances, preoperative optimisation 119
renal failure *31*, 33, 59, 60, 64, 115
renal function 52, 69
renal system 30–1
respiratory disease
  implications 61–4
  morbidity prediction 87
  preoperative optimisation 102–7
respiratory system
  examination 27–8
  history 26–7
responsible minority test 136
retinopathy, diabetic 32
rhabdomyolysis 22
rheumatoid arthritis 33, 69
  implications 67–8
risk
  defined 79
  indicators of 83–8
  quantifying 79–80
risk assessment 14, 79–88
  mathematical modelling 81–2
  steps in process of 80–1
  thromboembolic 24, *25*
routine screening 6–7
routine testing 36

salbutamol 104, 177
saline 108, 109, 114, 115, 120, 126
Saturday Clubs 178
schizophrenia 71
scoring systems 80–1
screening 5, 6–7
sectionalised consent 138–9
Sengstaken-Blakemore tube 118
sensitivity, test performance 39
sensory neuropathy 65
serum biochemistry 51–3
serum lipid profile 45
serum potassium 29, 99
serum urea 67
severity of illness 83–4
shunting 118, 119
sickle cell disease 33, 121–2
Sickledex test 121–2
Sidaway 137, 144
sinus bradycardia 98
sinus node dysfunction 99
sinus tachycardia 99
sleepiness 31
smoking 21, 61, 86, 106–7, 121
snoring 27
social practices 21
sodium 113, 114, 119
sodium citrate 30, 174, 179
sodium retention 31, 112
solids 150, 161
specificity, test performance 39–40
Spielberger Stait/Trait Inventory (STAI) 11
spinal haematomata 30
spirometry 102, 106
spironolactone 112, 119
sputum 27
standards, preanaesthetic care 8
state anxiety 10, 11
stenosis 101
steroids 13, 32, 33, 52, 73, 103, 104, 111, 112, 128, 179, *180*
stiff joint syndrome 65
streptokinase 124
stress 152
Strict Advanced Trauma Life Support (ATLS) protocols 17
succinylcholine 128, 129

sucralfate 125
sulphonylureas 32, 108
surgery
  CAD 96
  cardiac risk 86
  consent 143–4
surgical severity 37
suxamethonium 29, 70, 73, 157
sweating 112
systems-based risk assessment 84–8

tachyarrhythmias 24, 65, 99–100
tachycardia 21, 24, 99–100, 112, 150,
    166, 175
tachykinins 66
tachypnoca 21, 28
temazepam 168, 177
terbutaline 104
testing see preoperative testing
tetany 112, 115
theophyllines 104, 173
thiazide 115
thiopentone 165
thrombin time (TT) 122
thrombocytopenia 123
thromboembolic risk assessment 24,
    25
thromboembolism 24, 30, 106
thrombolytic agents 85
thymectomy 128
thyroid disease
  implications 65
  preoperative assessment 32, 52
  preoperative optimisation 110–11
thyrotoxicosis 65, 100
tourniquets 33

trait anxiety 10–11
tranquillisers 73
transvenous pacing 98
trauma 34
trimeprazine 178
tumours, gut 66

ulnar deviation 33
unconscious patients, consent 139–40
upper respiratory tract infection
    (URTI) 63–4, 105
uraemia 67, 125
uraemic cardiomyopathy 67
urea nitrogen 52

valvular heart disease 97, 101
vascular disease 44–5
vasodilators 96
ventricular arrhythmias 100–1
ventricular fibrillation 164
verapamil 72, 100
verbal consent 136
viral myocarditis 63
vitamin K 117, 118, 122
vomiting, postoperative 22
von Willebrand disease 122, 123,
    124–5

warfarin 123, 173
wheezing 27, 63
white blood cell count 50–1
workplace, risk assessment 79

x rays, pulmonary 50

zafirlukast 103